THE 14-DAY NEW KETO CLEANSE

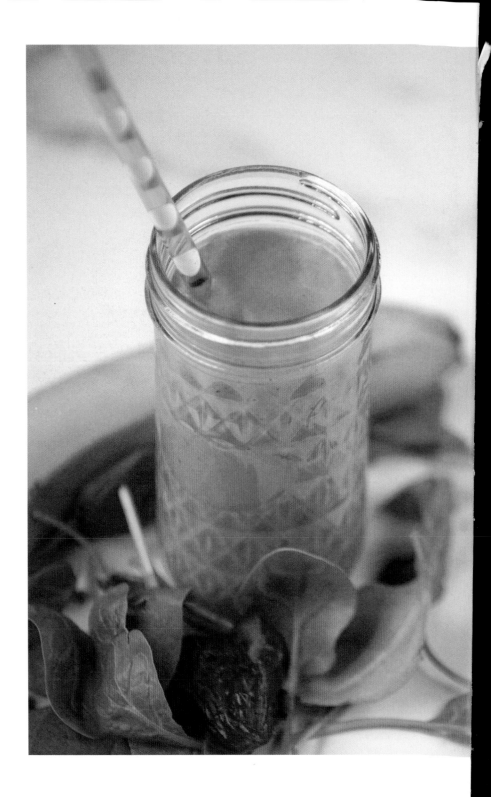

THE 14-DAY NEW KETO CLEANSE

Lose Up to 15 Pounds in 2 Weeks with Delicious Meals and Low-Sugar Smoothies

JJ SMITH

SIMON
ELEMENT

New York London Toronto Sydney New Delhi

**SIMON
ELEMENT**

An Imprint of Simon & Schuster, Inc.
1230 Avenue of the Americas
New York, NY 10020

First Simon Element trade paperback edition April 2022

SIMON ELEMENT is a trademark of Simon & Schuster, Inc.

For information about special discounts for bulk purchases, please contact Simon & Schuster Special Sales at 1-866-506-1949 or business@simonandschuster.com.

The Simon & Schuster Speakers Bureau can bring authors to your live event. For more information or to book an event, contact the Simon & Schuster Speakers Bureau at 1-866-248-3049 or visit our website at www.simonspeakers.com.

Interior design by Renato Stanisic

Manufactured in the United States of America

10 9 8 7 6 5 4 3 2 1

Library of Congress Cataloging-in-Publication Data has been applied for.

ISBN 978-1-6680-0446-3
ISBN 978-1-6680-0447-0 (ebook)

Medical Disclaimer

The author does not guarantee that any products or recommendations will provide you with the same benefits that she has achieved. You should seek a doctor and do your own research to determine if any of the products or recommendations made in this book by the author would work for you. Additionally, the author is not paid for recommending any books or products in this book.

While the author has made every effort to provide accurate product names and contact information, such as Internet addresses, at the time of publication, neither the publisher nor the author assumes responsibility for errors or changes that occur after publication. Additionally, the author does not have any control over products or websites associated with the products listed in this book or the content of those websites.

This book is sold with the understanding that neither the author nor publisher, Simon Element, is engaged in rendering any legal, accounting, financial, medical, or other professional advice. If legal, financial, or medical expertise is required, the services of a competent professional should be sought, as no one at Simon Element is a medical practitioner. The author and publisher shall have neither liability nor responsibility to any person, company, or entity with respect to any loss or damage caused directly or indirectly by the concepts, ideas, products, information, or suggestions presented in this book. By reading this book, you agree to be bound by the statements above.

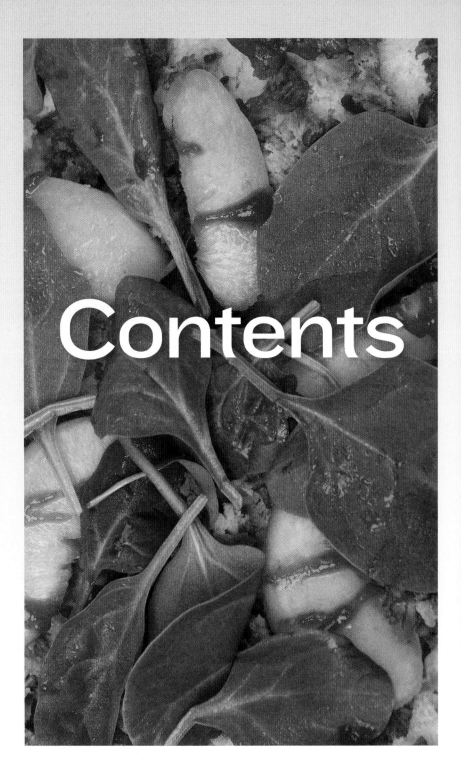

Contents

Important Note to Readers ix

Introduction 1

Chapter 1: What Is the 14-Day New Keto Cleanse? 11

Chapter 2: The Four Pillars of the New Keto Cleanse 21

Chapter 3: Getting Prepared/What to Expect
on the 14-Day New Keto Cleanse 41

Chapter 4: How to Do the 14-Day New Keto Cleanse 49

Chapter 5: The Keto Smoothie Recipes 63

Chapter 6: The Low-Carb, Fat-Burning
Meals and Snack Recipes 77

Chapter 7: JJ's Personal Tips for Success 139

Chapter 8: How to Continue Losing Weight
After the 14-Day New Keto Cleanse 147

Chapter 9: Frequently Asked Questions (FAQs) 155

Chapter 10: Testimonials 167

Chapter 11: Conclusion 183

Appendix: JJ's Top Ten Favorite Detox Methods 187

Important Note to Readers

The information contained in this book is for your education. It is not intended to diagnose, treat, or cure any medical condition or dispense medical advice. If you decide to follow the plan, you should seek the advice and counsel of a licensed health professional and then use your own judgment.

It is important to obtain proper medical advice before you make any decisions about nutrition, diet, supplements, or other health-related issues discussed in this book. Neither the author nor the publisher is qualified to provide medical, financial, or psychological advice or services. The reader should consult an appropriate health care professional before heeding any of the advice given in this book.

THE 14-DAY NEW KETO CLEANSE

Introduction

Congratulations on taking back control of your health and weight! *The 14-Day New Keto Cleanse* teaches you lessons on weight loss, health, metabolism, energy, and longevity. You can reset your body's chemistry to make weight loss easier and add healthier days to your life. My desire is that obesity, depression, disease, and fatigue all become a thing of the past. I believe you can and will take back control of your health and weight.

Battling excess weight can be one of the most frustrating, challenging, and emotionally draining experiences on earth. Many people struggle with a never-ending battle to lose weight and become healthy. Despite the numerous fad diets, skinny teas, and exercise regimens for weight loss, year after year, Americans continue to get bigger. The diet industry continues to grow larger and larger. The sad fact is that about 70 percent of Americans are obese and struggling to get to their goal weight.

The 14-Day New Keto Cleanse is a complete guide for healthy, fast weight loss. You will learn how to detox your body, improve your health, and get your body into fat-burning mode. Doing so will assist you in losing weight more easily. I will lay out the foundation for living a longer, healthier life. If you are really committed to bettering your health, this book will provide you with a detailed plan toward a life filled with improved health, energy, and the reversal of many diseases and ailments you may be dealing with.

The book will help you get into ketosis, or fat-burning mode. However, this book does not delve into the complicated science and chemistry behind ketosis. I don't want to confuse you with an overload of data. Instead, my approach is to present the information in plain, simple language, the same way I talk to my friends and family.

This book is specifically written for those who want a healthier version of keto, without all the side effects and long-term health challenges of the standard, high-fat keto diet. Thus, this is a practical guide for leveraging the principles of ketosis to help you get to your goal weight once and for all.

This book is for you if you

- struggle with losing weight and keeping it off;
- struggle with belly fat, even when you lose weight from other parts of your body;
- need improved mental clarity and energy levels;
- are starting to feel old and tired and need to feel healthier;
- want to cut down on the number of doctor visits;
- long for the day you wake up without pain and fatigue; or
- dream of having the energy to play with your children and grandchildren.

Is This Your Story?

I want to tell you the story of Casey. Casey's health resembles that of most Americans, particularly as they age. Like many, Casey thought she would age slowly, one day at a time, hardly noticing any change. But as the years went by, Casey could feel and see changes in her face and body. She began to realize there was something accelerating her aging. "Why the accelerated aging and weight gain?" she thought. One simple answer: chronic inflammation.

What is chronic inflammation? When cells are damaged within the body, inflammation is your body's natural response to an injury or threat. Chronic inflammation puts your body into an emergency crisis for a prolonged period, eventually leading to other health problems. If left untreated, chronic inflammation, also known as systemic inflammation, can persist for months or even for years. Oftentimes, underlying conditions such as autoimmune diseases, toxin buildup, or infection can cause chronic inflammation to stick around longer. When chronic inflammation lingers too long, the immune system continues pumping out white blood cells that prolong the process, making the inflammation last even longer.

When inflammation is present, even those with the most disciplined eating and exercise routines may find it difficult to lose weight. Research shows that weight gain is associated with increased inflammation in the body. Many studies show that inflammation is a common underlying factor in most major degenerative diseases such as hypertension, cancer, heart disease, and diabetes. Studies also show that inflammation can cause weight gain and make it difficult to lose any weight at all.

A major benefit of following the 14-Day New Keto Cleanse is reduced inflammation, which leads to easier weight loss and improved health. Simply put, until inflammation is addressed, you cannot successfully lose weight and keep it off.

Casey's clothes began to fit snugly—her baggy sweatpants

were fitting like skinny jeans. Her stamina and energy levels began to decline as well. Casey would begin a new diet, and in most cases, the diet would help her easily lose fifteen to twenty pounds. However, the weight would always come back. Not only that, but the diets that had always worked for her in the past were becoming less effective and failing to work as quickly as they once had. This yo-yo dieting also left her metabolism wrecked and her body chemically changed. As she gained weight, millions of cells in her body stretched and swelled with fluid buildup. As she lost weight, some of the fluid left her cells, but not all of it. So, the cells became modified, leaving an altered body chemistry, which caused her health to decline and the weight to increase.

Every time Casey began another diet, it altered her cellular chemistry in a negative way. To lose weight, Casey would undergo extreme calorie reduction, but that would become less and less effective. Extreme diets often require you to lower your calorie intake, but if you don't provide your body with adequate nutrition, it will go into starvation mode and begin to hold on to fat for future use. As a survival mechanism, fat cells respond to starvation by holding on to the fat they already have, making it more difficult to shed fat in the long run.

So as the years went by, Casey continued to pack on the pounds. More and more of her clothes were being thrown into the box called "When I lose weight"! However, she needed more boxes year after year, as there had been no pounds lost. It was devastating to know that she had so much personal and professional success in other areas of her life but couldn't find a way to get slim and healthy. Years of trying to lose weight had made her feel weak, frustrated, and dejected.

Casey continued to follow every new fad diet that came out, especially if a friend or coworker had experienced success with it. She would always begin her new diet with much enthusiasm and commitment, only to gain the weight back in the end. Casey, who was deeply involved in her church, even used her faith to deal with cravings and the desire to eat. She thought she just needed more prayer and more discipline to fight off the feelings of hunger and boredom while dieting. But with every failed attempt, Casey felt increasingly frustrated. With each failed attempt, her belief that she could actually achieve her goal weight diminished.

Anytime Casey ate less and reduced her caloric intake, she became sad and depressed. Without knowing it, she was dialing down her metabolism at the cellular level, making fat burning even more difficult. Casey also learned that extreme dieting was likely the cause of chronic inflammation in her body, as diagnosed by her doctor. Chronic inflammation not only caused Casey to gain weight but also likely was aging her brain and body, making her memory and mental sharpness things of the past. Inflammation was also making her body feel old, with achy joints and knees. If Casey didn't make a change, she would have a difficult time losing weight with loss of vitality and energy.

Casey wondered if extreme calorie cutting was the only way to lose weight. The answer is no, as there are many ways to lose weight, including

- reducing the number of calories consumed (but not extreme calorie reduction),
- detoxing and healing your body,

- balancing your hormones, and/or
- revving up your metabolism.

Imagine a weight loss plan that does all those things to allow you to get to your goal weight faster and make weight loss easier! Well, you have the solution in your hands. It's called the 14-Day New Keto Cleanse, and it accomplishes all of the above. On the New Keto Cleanse, you focus on reducing carbs, detoxing the body, balancing your hormones, and revving up your metabolism.

The New Keto Cleanse is *not* the standard keto diet but a fresh approach to keto that combines the nutritional benefits of green smoothies with the sweet state of ketosis to provide maximum fat loss. By following the ketogenic nutritional guidelines, combined with intermittent fasting, you can significantly speed up the fat-burning process, helping you achieve your health and weight-loss goals more rapidly.

The New Keto Cleanse uses low-sugar keto smoothies and low-carb, fat-burning meals to help the body get into ketosis (fat-burning mode) so your metabolism stays revved up. This meal plan also helps you detox with green smoothies. By eating blended foods (green smoothies), you are giving your digestive system a break while freeing up your body to do some repair work. When you drink green smoothies, your body will begin to do some much needed cleansing and healing. Finally, this meal plan will assist in reducing inflammation to help reverse disease and slow aging. An added benefit is that you also address hormonal imbalances, such as insulin resistance, which can occur when there is chronic inflammation in the body.

The new keto approach I recommend involves a healthier

version of keto, combined with intermittent fasting and some minor physical activity. I will not only provide general guidelines for the correct amounts of carbs, proteins, and fats but also focus on high-quality, nutrient-dense foods to ensure that you get the proper nutrition to heal and fuel your body. Many keto plans focus on extreme carb cutting and high fats. However, extreme carb cutting is not always healthy in the long run and often causes rebound weight gain. Some keto plans don't always focus on quality nutrients in foods, either. However, I will focus on a healthier keto, combined with intermittent fasting, which is the most powerful weapon you can use to achieve your health goals.

This will not be as hard as you think, because when you combine a healthier form of keto with intermittent fasting, you can stop cravings and reduce your appetite between meals. So that you can stay on this plan for life, you will have the freedom to eat savory, delicious meals without cravings and hunger.

Why I Created the 14-Day New Keto Cleanse

Over the last eight years, I have coached tens of thousands of people to help them lose over ten million pounds.

Here is how it all started for me. A few years ago, after years of clean, healthy eating and detoxing, I became terribly ill. I was bedridden. It turned out I had gotten mercury poisoning from my silver dental fillings! I had high levels of mercury in my brain, gut, liver, and kidneys. I couldn't get out of bed for two months. And when I did, just making the bed required that I lie back down to rest! My health, energy, and motivation were at an all-time low.

After a long and slow recovery, I decided I needed to do

something to get my health and energy back, as well as lose the twenty pounds I had gained while bedridden. After learning how raw greens can heal the body, I created my 10-Day Green Smoothie Cleanse. Also, already an advocate of detoxing, I knew I needed to rid my body of the waste and toxins that had accumulated as a result of the mercury poisoning.

Once I created the 10-Day Green Smoothie Cleanse, I asked my community of friends and family if they would join and support me. My goal was to get ten people to say yes. I was pleasantly surprised to find that about one hundred of them wanted to do it! I created a Facebook group to keep us all motivated. Because the results, which we shared through pictures and testimonials, were so phenomenal, in less than two months about ten thousand people had joined the Facebook group and committed to doing the cleanse with us. In just ten days, folks were losing ten to fifteen pounds, getting energized, reversing health conditions, and feeling better than they had in years. Today, the Facebook group has over 850,000 members supporting one another along their weight-loss journey.

When I completed my first cleanse, I lost eleven pounds. My energy was high, my skin was radiant, and my digestion and bloating had improved. I felt renewed and motivated again! Before I began the cleanse, I had been taking twenty-four supplements a day to help my body recover from mercury poisoning. Since completing the cleanse, I have been taking only four supplements per day and have such a positive outlook on my health that I now have the energy to focus on my life dreams and goals. I learned that green smoothies are a great way to give the body the nutrition it needs not only to keep it healthy and vibrant but also to nourish the spark of life within it.

Fast-forward to today. Ten million pounds have been lost on the Green Smoothie Cleanse, which I codified into a book, the number-one *New York Times* bestseller *10-Day Green Smoothie Cleanse*. The book's techniques are so successful and the word of mouth about the diet so organic that the book has stayed on the *New York Times* bestseller list for fifty-two consecutive weeks, and I now have close to three million followers/fans on social media.

Over the last year, more and more of my followers were asking whether they should do the keto diet. How could they fit their beloved green smoothies into the keto guidelines, given all the fruit in them? How could they do the keto diet without all the high fat and rebound weight gain? Due to more and more people asking me questions about the keto diet, I decided to create a more nutritional version of it that allowed you to still detox while also maximizing fat burning in the body.

While the 10-Day Green Smoothie Cleanse is a very effective detox that will jump-start weight loss, the 14-Day New Keto Cleanse is designed more specifically for fat burning and sustainable weight loss. It has low-sugar keto smoothies, low-carb, fat-burning meals, and other lifestyle habits that put the body into fat-burning mode! The 14-Day New Keto Cleanse is an effective weight-loss plan that will help you burn fat faster, all while enjoying delicious meals.

Here's why you should have confidence that this plan will work for you:

- This plan is well tested. I have successfully tested the 14-Day New Keto Cleanse with tens of thousands of people around the world who can attest that it works (see testimonial chapter).

- I've made the plan easy to follow with a day-by-day regimen detailing what to eat each day, with very quick and easy meal plans.
- The low-sugar keto smoothies still allow you to detox using keto-friendly ingredients that are lower in carbs and sugar than the ingredients in traditional green smoothies.
- The low-carb fat-burning meals are flavorful, delicious, nutrient-dense, and filling so you will stay satisfied during this plan.

I know how much courage it takes to begin a new life and a new relationship with food. I support you and encourage you in your efforts. I suggest you read this book just for understanding at first and then reread it with a mind to take action and begin your journey. Get a copy for a family member and friend so that you all can encourage and support one another through this life-changing transformation. Your family, friends, and I will be here to guide you along and support you. In fact, support will be very helpful to you on this journey. Join 850,000 others who get free support from me and my team on a daily basis on our Facebook page at https://www.facebook.com/groups/Green.Smoothie.Cleanse/. You are not alone. We will do this together. Let your journey begin today.

Will you join me in this journey to heal the body, lose weight, and increase energy levels? By doing this, you will never have to worry about weight again. This is an amazing way to transform your body in just fourteen days. So, get ready to start your 14-Day New Keto Cleanse today!

CHAPTER 1

What Is the 14-Day New Keto Cleanse?

The New Keto Cleanse is a fresh approach to getting into ketosis. It uses low-sugar keto smoothies along with low-carb, fat-burning meals to detox, reduce cravings, and burn fat faster. To help you speed up the fat-burning process and achieve your health and weight-loss goals more rapidly, I provide guidelines for getting into ketosis that include delicious meals, intermittent fasting, and minor physical activity.

What Is Ketosis (Keto)?

Our bodies are natural fat-burning machines, but due to the consumption of processed high-sugar foods, we have become dependent on carbs to supply us with energy. To lose weight, we need to reset our hormones and create the right environment for the body to burn stored fat—a process known as ketosis.

Ketosis is when the body starts converting stored fat into ketones to use as fuel for the cells.

So, what are ketones? When your fuel comes from fat, your body makes molecules called ketones. Your cells produce ketones when they're fed fat. When the ketones swim throughout the body and your bloodstream, they fuel your cells with a source of energy that is steady and strong all day.

Ketones show up in your body when your cells use fat for energy. So, it's important to eat fat to burn fat. The one food that doesn't raise insulin levels is fat. By eating high levels of healthy fats, you help the body get into ketosis faster and stay full longer. So, lowering the carbs and increasing the fats is the way to get into ketosis.

Keep in mind that you cannot get into ketosis with high insulin levels. Remember that eating carbs increases blood sugar levels, which increases insulin levels. High insulin levels prevent you from getting into ketosis.

How long will it take to get into ketosis? It depends on the individual. Some folks can enter ketosis overnight, while others can take a month or longer to get into this fat-burning mode. Scientists say the shift from using glucose to breaking down stored fat as a source of energy usually begins over two to four days of eating fewer than twenty to fifty grams of carbohydrates per day. However, everyone is different, and this time frame may be longer for some.

This healthier version of the keto plan focuses on high-quality, nutrient-dense foods, ensuring that you get the proper nutrition to heal and fuel your body as you get into ketosis. Dirty keto is when your main focus is staying in ketosis, regardless of the quality of the nutrients you consume. As an example, dirty keto might mean you eat saturated fats such as bacon or fast food just to ensure you get your protein and fats in. A healthier version of keto, though, focuses on eating healthy fats, such as monounsaturated fats and polyunsaturated fats, which include olive oil, medium-chain triglyceride (MCT) oil, avocados, wild-caught salmon, nuts, seeds, and so on.

Reasons Why You Can't Get into Ketosis

When you first begin this program, you'll be focused on getting your body into ketosis. If you struggle to do so, or if you have struggled to get into ketosis in the past, there could be many reasons why. Here are the top four reasons folks can't get into ketosis and what they can do about it.

You're eating too many carbs. Most people can get into ketosis by keeping their net carbs under thirty grams per day. However, for some, the threshold may have to be even lower, at twenty grams net carbs per day. Many of us deal with sneaky carbs hidden in processed foods, so be sure to read nutritional labels to ensure you are indeed staying at that low level of carbs per day.

You haven't addressed toxins in the body. Toxic overload is a common reason folks struggle to get into ketosis. The more toxins you take in or get exposed to every day, the more toxins you store in your body's fat cells. Toxins stored in fat cells are difficult to get rid of through dieting alone. It's always important to address the toxins in your fat cells. The body can burn fat cells, but it cannot burn the toxins in those cells. To get rid of them, you have to detox your body. One of the reasons the keto smoothies are an important part of this program is that they help to flush toxins out of the body, making fat loss easier.

You haven't learned to manage electrolytes. Understanding electrolytes is critical on this program. When you lower carbs, you will release water, causing your kidneys to release more sodium. Sodium, an electrolyte, throws off the balance of other key electrolytes, such as potassium and magnesium. If you don't replenish these electrolytes, you will experience fatigue, headaches, brain fog, and trouble getting into ketosis. Replenishing those electrolytes generally solves this problem.

You lack sleep and have too much stress. Yes, not getting enough sleep and living a stressful life will keep you out of ketosis. When you lack sleep or are stressed, your body releases cortisol, which causes fat to be stored in the belly. So, the short story is that high cortisol levels increase belly fat. When cortisol levels are high, glucose levels rise and ketones drop, which will make it difficult to stay in ketosis.

What Makes This the "New" Keto?

Traditional keto diets are typically nutrient deficient because of the focus on fats, protein, and very low carb intake as opposed to quality nutrition. However, this New Keto Cleanse seeks nutritional ketosis; this gives you a macro nutritional boost focusing on high-quality, nutrient-dense foods to ensure you get the adequate nutrition to not only burn fat but also to heal and fuel the body as well.

There are five reasons this plan is a more nutritional, healthier version of keto:

Focuses on healthy fats: Some keto plans allow you to eat many high-fat foods, but not all fat is good fat. Too many people following the keto lifestyle eat too much saturated and trans fat, both of which are known to raise cholesterol, promote plaque deposits, and eventually clog your arteries and lead to heart disease. Although the keto diet is a high-fat diet, the majority of the fats should be healthy fats, which are monounsaturated and polyunsaturated fats. These healthy fats are linked to lower blood pressure, healthier blood sugar levels, and less inflammation in the body. They include avocado, wild-caught salmon, olives, nuts and seeds, olive oil, MCT oil, and coconut butter. These healthy fats raise your "good" cholesterol levels, so feel free to enjoy them. You will want to limit your intake of trans fats and saturated fat, as they can increase your "bad" cholesterol and put you at risk of heart disease. Examples of trans fats and saturated fats to limit include red meat, fried foods, vegetable oils including canola oil, and margarine.

Keto smoothies: One of the reasons the keto smoothies are an important of this program is because green smoothies help detox and flush toxins out of the body, making fat loss easier. Green smoothies have an incredibly powerful ability to detox the body while also giving your body the quality nutrition it needs. Vitamins, minerals, and other nutrients will be absorbed by your body more efficiently, allowing your cells to become like new as you begin to look and feel younger. Green smoothies are filled with chlorophyll, which is similar in structure to the hemoglobin in human blood. So every time you drink a green smoothie, it's like receiving a blood transfusion. They are a potent cleansing method for the body. The standard keto diet doesn't include keto smoothies, but they are an important and powerful aspect of this program.

Intermittent fasting: Significantly cutting carbs is one way to get into ketosis, as done in the standard keto diet. Another way is through fasting. Intermittent fasting accelerates the process of getting into ketosis. Intermittent fasting is an eating pattern where you alternate between periods of eating and fasting. I discuss intermittent fasting in great detail in the next chapter, because intermittent fasting is a key aspect of this New Keto Cleanse.

No extreme carb cutting: Unlike the strict keto diet, there will be no extreme carb cutting. Eating extremely low carbs for long periods of time can lead to eventual weight rebound where people gain all the weight back, plus some. Additionally, people underestimate how difficult it is to stick to a diet with extremely low carbohydrates. In the standard keto diet, dieters try to stay away from healthy fruits and vegetables because they fear their carb content. However, these carbs are healthy whole foods that are nutrient-packed and fiber-filled, make your diet nutritionally sound, and also help you avoid constipation.

Sustainable for life: There is no need to "go off" this new keto plan. When most follow the traditional keto diet, it is a short-term plan, without any guidelines for long-term weight loss. However, the real goal is to keep the weight off. With the balance of low-carb, healthy meals, keto smoothies, and intermittent fasting, you can continue to enjoy this plan for life since it's not too restrictive or unsafe. So, the key benefits of ketosis, such as reduced inflammation, autophagy, etc., can continue for as long as you live because you never have to go off this new keto plan.

I'm confident that this "new" keto cleanse is the most powerful weapon you can use to achieve your health and weight-loss goals.

Why You Don't Need Prolonged Ketosis to Have Success on This Program

Eating a low amount of carbohydrates over the long term is a good thing for your health and body. It will help with fat loss and overall health and energy. However, there is no need to pursue a constant state of ketosis, where your body is continually burning its own fat for fuel. This will become unsustainable, because eventually your body will have no more fat to burn. This program will allow you to achieve a long-term healthy lifestyle without needing to be in a constant state of ketosis.

Ketosis is great for burning fat fast, but if you don't come out of it, it will burn through all your excess body fat and then begin to shut off other bodily functions, which could be fatal. Additionally, if you stay in ketosis for too long, your body will sense that your fat reserves are depleting and, as a survival tactic, will slow down fat burning over time, which also slows your metabolism.

Prolonged ketosis can lead to hormonal imbalances such as hypothyroidism, which slows your metabolism. Another hormonal imbalance that can occur with prolonged ketosis is leptin resistance, which prevents the signals the stomach sends to let you know when to stop eating from getting to the brain.

The good news is that to get the benefits of this plan, you don't have to fixate on being in ketosis.

Benefits of the 14-Day New Keto Cleanse

Fat loss

This plan wins at healthy, sustainable fat loss. People are surprised at how easily they can burn fat when they follow this plan. One reason this plan works is that the hormonal changes that occur while on the New Keto Cleanse improve your metabolic function. This allows your body to burn more fat and stay in fat-burning mode.

Improved mental clarity and brain function

You can expect improved brain function as well as more mental clarity and energy. If you experience brain fog, which means you are unable to think clearly and concentrate, you can expect that to improve while following this plan. The reason you may experience brain fog is because of blood sugar spikes. The solution to avoiding brain fog is intermittent fasting, which allows you to skip breakfast and minimize the amount of food you eat all day. This will result in fewer blood sugar spikes and less brain fog. Intermittent fasting also stimulates the growth of new brain neurons, which help to develop and preserve a healthy brain.

Clearer, radiant skin

Healthy, glowing skin results from this plan. After the first ketone is produced, skin redness and inflammation slowly fade and new skin cells are produced. The most noticeable improvement in your skin begins to show one to two months after being in ketosis. It happens because you're reducing inflammation. Skin problems such as acne are caused by inflammation. Any skin cells that were formed during ketosis were made in the absence of inflammation. So, when you stop the inflammation, more youthful and radiant skin can appear a few weeks later.

Improved sleep

Expect an improvement in sleep quality and duration. In the beginning, due to low levels of serotonin, this plan may cause interrupted sleep and insomnia. In the long term, however, you can expect deeper sleep, including improved rapid eye movement (REM) sleep. REM sleep is the stage of sleep where most dreaming takes place. REM sleep also improves mental concentration and mood, so it enhances your overall quality of life.

Reduced risk of diabetes

As you become overweight or obese, you increase the risk of type 2 diabetes. There is a correlation between weight gain and insulin resistance, which leads to type 2 diabetes. When you become insulin resistant, your pancreas does not produce enough insulin to keep your blood sugar levels under control. High blood sugar levels increase the risk of developing type 2 diabetes. Maybe someone reading this has already had this happen to them. However, the good news is that the New Keto Cleanse lowers insulin resistance so that your blood sugar levels drop, lowering your insulin levels.

Less inflammation

This plan has many anti-inflammatory benefits. Studies show that the state of ketosis provides a metabolic shift that reduces inflammation. When cells are damaged on the inside of the body, inflammation is your body's natural response to the injury or threat. If left untreated, chronic inflammation, also known as systemic inflammation, can persist for months or years. Chronic inflammation puts your body into an emergency crisis for a prolonged period of time, which eventually leads to other health problems. Many studies show that inflammation is a common underlying factor in most major degenerative diseases such as hypertension, cancer, heart disease, and diabetes. So, reducing inflammation will not only help with weight loss but also reduce the chance of degenerative diseases.

Increased autophagy

Autophagy, another major benefit of this plan, is the body's way of cleaning out damaged cells to regenerate newer, healthier cells. Autophagy decreases inflammation and improves organ function. By killing infected cells before they can spread and infect other cells, autophagy is extremely important for our immune system function.

CHAPTER 2

The Four Pillars of the New Keto Cleanse

The 14-Day New Keto Cleanse consists of four pillars that will help you get a healthier body in two weeks, with less body fat, a slimmer waistline, and more radiant energy.

Keto Smoothies

By now you know that green smoothies are good for your health! Green smoothies are surprisingly simple, consisting of raw organic fruit, raw organic leafy greens, and water. Despite their simplicity, green smoothies provide a ton of nutritional benefits that lead to a healthier lifestyle. These benefits include weight loss, increased energy, reduction in food cravings, clearer skin, and much more.

However, when I transitioned to a healthier version of keto, I couldn't enjoy the traditional green smoothies I am known for. This is because of the high volume of fruit in them. What always made green smoothies taste good was the sweet fruit. So, I became determined to find a way to make keto-friendly smoothies taste great, without all the sugar.

A low-sugar diet will help you avoid many health issues and live a much a healthier lifestyle. Eating too much sugar has many negative health effects, with the most obvious being

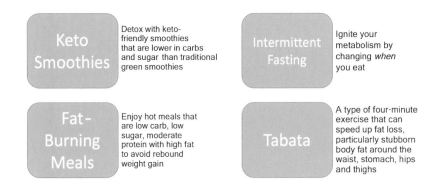

weight gain. Excess sugar in your diet causes high insulin levels, alters your metabolism, and causes the extra calories to turn into belly fat.

When you eat sugar, it gets stored in your liver in the form of glycogen. When your liver is overloaded with sugar, it begins to expand, and when it's maxed out, the glycogen is expelled in the form of fatty acids. This excess fat is deposited in areas such as the belly, butt, thighs, and hips. The danger is when fatty acids end up in our major organs, such as the heart and the kidneys.

Sugary foods (candy, cakes, pies, muffins, and sodas) and other refined, starchy carbohydrates cause a rapid rise in insulin levels, which results in excess fat in the body. When food is eaten, the body breaks it down into glucose so it can be used as fuel. Insulin is the hormone that sends glucose out of the blood and into the tissue cells for use as energy. When excess glucose remains in the blood, insulin levels stay high. Chronically elevated insulin can cause both fat storage and more inflammation in the body. High insulin levels are a signal to the body to store extra calories as fat and to refrain from burning fat.

Research has also shown that a high-sugar diet causes cancer cells to multiply rapidly. An important study published in the medical journal *Cancer Research* by a team at the University of California, Los Angeles, found that while sugar of any kind offered sustenance to cancer cells, fructose played a key role in the cells' proliferation. That means that cancer spreads more quickly on a high-fructose diet.

If you want to look and feel your best while also avoiding long-term health issues, a low-sugar diet is the way to go.

After weeks of trial and error, I finally cracked the code on what ingredients I could use to make the green smoothies taste creamy and delicious while staying low-sugar as well. That's what I've included with this plan: keto smoothies with the right taste, texture, and variety. You will detox with keto-friendly smoothies that are lower in carbs and lower in sugar than traditional green smoothies. Each recipe is designed to be under fifteen net carbs per serving. I've combined the nutritional benefits of green smoothies with the fat-burning benefits of keto to allow you to detox, reduce cravings, and lose weight in just fourteen days.

Keto Smoothie Core Ingredients

Keto smoothies are nutrient rich and have some key ingredients you'll be using throughout this cleanse. There are the core ingredients, which are low in sugar and low in carbs:

- **Spinach:** Spinach is one of the primary ingredients in any green or keto smoothie. Spinach is the mildest-tasting green. You can barely taste the spinach in a smoothie. Spinach is packed with nutrients such as magnesium, potassium, calcium, iron, vitamin C, and soluble fiber. The most commonly used spinach in these recipes is baby spinach.

- **Unsweetened almond milk:** For this cleanse, you will often see unsweetened vanilla almond milk used as the liquid. It is a lactose-free and soy-free milk substitute that is made primarily of ground almonds and water. It's also low on the glycemic index, making it a great choice for people who want to avoid sugar. If you are allergic to almond milk, you can use any unsweetened nut, seed, or soy milk.

- **Flaxseeds:** For this cleanse, I use ground flaxseeds, which are high in fiber and omega-3 fatty acids in addition to being a rich source of some vitamins and minerals. Flaxseeds are also called a functional food, which means that a person can eat them to simply boost their health. Flaxseeds don't have to be stored in a refrigerator, but do keep them in an airtight container.

- **Almond butter:** Almond butter is one of the most nutrient-dense nut butters available. It contains much more calcium, magnesium, manganese, and phosphorus than peanut butter. It's also high in vitamin E, an essential antioxidant that is great for eye and heart health. Almond butter is also high in fiber and low in saturated fat, which could help to improve cholesterol panels.

- **Avocado:** I am no fan of avocados, but luckily, they have no taste in a smoothie. They also make a smoothie thick and creamy. They are nutritious and heart healthy. They are loaded with healthy fats, fiber, and various important nutrients. Avocados are a great source of healthy monounsaturated fat, which makes you more satisfied and tends to fill you up as well. An alternative to avocados would be Greek yogurt, with less than five grams of sugar.

- **MCT oil:** A popular ingredient in the keto community is MCT oil. Medium-chain triglycerides (MCTs) are fats found in foods such as coconut oil. They are metabolized differently than the long-chain triglycerides (LCTs) found in other foods. Because MCTs are digested more quickly than LCTs, they get to be used as energy first, and many find that they improve energy, brain function, and mental clarity. MCT oil also won't change the flavor of a smoothie.

- **Coconut oil:** Coconut oil is made by pressing the fat from the white "meat" inside the giant nut. The majority of its calories come from saturated fat. But the good news is that coconut oil's saturated fat is made up mostly of medium-chain triglycerides, or MCTs, which are explained above.

- **Plant-based protein powder:** I use a plant-based protein powder in all my smoothies to increase my protein intake, help me stay full longer, and keep my metabolism revved up. The protein can make the smoothie taste slightly pasty, so I use small amounts to avoid affecting the taste of the keto smoothie. Feel free to use any nondairy, plant-based protein powder, such as rice, soy, or hemp protein, but not whey protein powder, which is made from cow's milk.

- **Low-sugar fruits:** On a standard keto diet, many fruits are off limits. However, some fruits, such as berries, are low in sugar and can fit into this healthier keto plan. As an example, strawberries have five net carbs in half a cup. So, you will find limited use of some fruit in this plan.

- **Stevia:** With traditional green smoothies, stevia is often not needed due to the amount of fruit in them. However, with keto smoothies, stevia or another natural sweetener (e.g., monk fruit) is often required if it's included in the recipe. The way to think about sweeteners is how much they cause insulin spikes because that determines how much they will cause fat storage in the body. Foods are given glycemic index (GI) ratings according to how much they cause insulin spikes. Stevia and monk fruit are a 0 (which is ideal). Agave is a 20. Honey is about a 30. Brown sugar and raw sugar are both a 65. And refined white sugar is an 80.

- **Vanilla yogurt:** Although frozen fruit will keep your smoothies thick and frosty, with keto smoothies, you use less or no fruit, and yogurt becomes a good substitute. Yogurt is also a great protein source. However, many on the market are high in sugar. So, I recommend a low-sugar yogurt that helps provide the creamy texture in a smoothie. I use yogurt in a few of my keto smoothies.

Low-Carb, Fat-Burning Meals

Everything—from what you eat to what you drink—affects your weight. That's why it's important to eat foods that not only taste good but also help to shed fat.

The 14-Day Keto Cleanse includes hot meals that are low-carb and low-sugar, with moderate protein and healthy fats to ensure maximum fat loss. This cleanse lays out a more balanced approach to eating good carbs, healthy fats, and lean protein, which prevents rebounds in weight gain. It also provides forty new recipes (eleven keto smoothies and twenty-nine meal and snack recipes). These recipes include *fat-burning meals* that are especially designed to promote fat loss by revving up the metabolism, reducing appetite, and reducing overall sugar-carb intake. Eating these low-carb, fat-burning meals can help you

- burn fat faster,
- rev up your metabolism,
- feel fuller longer, and
- build muscle that naturally burns more calories than fat.

When a person adds these fat-burning meals to their diet, they can burn fat and lose weight over time.

You will enjoy this healthy eating plan, which will help you balance hormones, decrease hunger, regulate your metabolism, and remove toxins that lead to chronic disease. The ingredients in the fat-burning meal recipes include lean proteins, good carbs, and healthy fats.

What Are Macronutrients, and Why Do They Matter?

When you first begin this program, you will want to learn about macronutrients, also called *macros*, for they are the major nutritional elements that make up the caloric content of your food. Macros are the three categories of food that fuel our bodies. There's a whole bunch of technical science that I could detail, but my goal is to keep this simple. All food falls into one of these three categories: proteins, fats, and carbohydrates.

Many people calculate and track their macros on the keto

diet, but with this plan, I will provide a more efficient way for you to monitor your macros without the tediousness of macro calculators.

The typical keto diet consists of

- 5 percent carbs,
- 20 percent proteins, and
- 75 percent fats.

This healthier version of keto is more flexible, consisting of

- 10 percent carbs,
- 20 percent proteins, and
- 70 percent fats (focusing on healthy fats).

Proteins

On this plan, you need to consume a moderate amount of protein. Protein provides the building blocks to form nearly every tissue in your body, including muscle. Research shows that moderate protein on keto diets is perfectly compatible with weight loss, ketone production, and other health benefits.

As a general guideline, *moderate* is between three and six ounces (about as much as you can fit in the palm of your hand) of protein per meal, but the amounts may vary depending upon certain factors. As an example, if you work out or are younger, you will need more protein, so feel free to increase protein intake. Be sure you consume high-quality proteins such as fish, poultry, or eggs.

Fats

Seventy percent of your calories should be from healthy fats. This might seem like a lot of fat, but what is important is that healthy fats fuel the body. Examples of healthy fats include olive oil, MCT oil, wild-caught salmon, and nuts and seeds. Fat is the most filling and satisfying macronutrient. It also triggers insulin the least. Stable insulin levels prevent blood sugar spikes and keep your body from storing extra fat.

Adding more fat to your meals can help you fast longer during intermittent fasting. If you're feeling hungry after a meal, feel free to adjust fats upward. Over time, as you continue on this program, hunger and cravings will be reduced naturally. However, be sure not to overdo it with fats. You could overwhelm the gallbladder and begin to feel symptoms such as bloating, nausea, burping, and dull pain in your right shoulder.

One of the common mistakes people make when following the keto lifestyle is eating too much saturated and trans fats. Although the new keto diet is a high-fat diet, the majority of the fats should be healthy fats, which are monounsaturated fat and polyunsaturated fats. They raise your "good" cholesterol levels, so feel free to enjoy them. You will want to limit your intake of trans fats and saturated fats because they can increase your "bad" cholesterol and put you at risk of heart disease. Examples of trans fats and saturated fats to limit include red meats, fried foods, vegetable oils, canola oil, and margarine.

Carbs

Healthy carbs on this program include non-starchy veggies, salads, and green leafy vegetables. The goal is to make sure your foods are as low as possible in carbs, sugar, and starch. Honestly, restricting carbs is going to be the most challenging aspect of this program, but it's nonnegotiable if you want results. Keep in mind that low carbs means low sugar, which means low blood sugar, which means low insulin. Low insulin means you're in fat-burning mode. This is how you will get into ketosis. This is the most important thing you need to understand about this program.

Which Are the Best Macros for You?

The typical keto diet requires that you calculate and track your macros, and there are many keto macro calculators on the Internet. They will factor in your height, weight, activity levels, etc., to recommend the keto macros most ideal for you.

However, a simpler way to do this is to monitor your net carbs with each meal and enjoy a moderate amount of protein and a high level of healthy fats.

Net carbs are the carbohydrates in food that you cannot digest and use for energy. To calculate net carbs, you take the total carbs and subtract the fiber and sugar alcohols. Because fiber is a carbohydrate our body cannot digest, it passes through our digestive system unaltered. Also, sugar alcohols such as xylitol and erythritol are also indigestible, so they can be deducted from the total carb count as well. An example would be if the nutritional label says that total carbs are fourteen grams, dietary fiber is four grams, and sugar alcohols are six grams, then the net carbs are four grams. Many products now provide the net carbs on the nutritional label as well.

For weight loss, many recommend staying under twenty net carbs per day on the standard keto diet. However, this extreme restriction of carbs ultimately results in rebounds in weight gain and is not sustainable in the long run. Additionally, many have too many cravings and give in to temptation when trying to be too strict and stay under twenty grams of net carbs. So many can enjoy twenty to thirty net carbs per day and are still able to achieve their weight-loss goals. You could measure your blood ketones for a period of time to verify that up to thirty grams of net carbs per day still allows you to be successful on the program. However, it is not required to get great results.

What Is Intermittent Fasting?

Significantly cutting carbs is one way to get into ketosis. Another way is through fasting. Intermittent fasting accelerates the process of getting into ketosis. There are various forms of fasting, and there is a right way and a wrong way to fast to get the body into a state of ketosis. In fact, complete fasting with no food is unnecessary and can even be dangerous for people with diabetes, chronic kidney disease, and other health conditions.

Fasting allows you to feed, or fuel, your body with your own fat. Once you begin fasting, your body will first burn quickly through your glucose stores. Then, in less than twenty-four hours, your body will begin using stored body fat for fuel. Fat burning typically begins after twelve hours of fasting and then escalates between sixteen and twenty-four hours of fasting, as the body begins to produce ketones.

Intermittent fasting is an approach to eating where you switch between a period of time where you eat (an eating window) and a period of time that you don't eat (a fasting window). During the eating window, you eat normally, as you have no restrictions on which foods you can eat. However, the healthier you eat, the more dramatic your results will be. During the fasting window, you are not allowed to consume any food—no calories. You should, though, drink plenty of water and enjoy black coffee and teas during the fasting window.

Intermittent fasting is not about counting calories but rather about timing your eating. It does not focus on which foods to eat but rather when you should eat them. The whole point of intermittent fasting is to prevent the body from producing insulin—therefore, no food should be consumed during the fasting time. It is not a diet. It is an eating pattern to reduce your blood sugar, turn on your fat-burning hormones, and use your stored fats as fuel so that you lose weight faster.

With intermittent fasting, you will first notice more hunger. Once your body adjusts to daily fasting, your insulin levels will lower, and your brain will stop sending signals that you need to eat. In other words, the longer you maintain a regular fasting method, the easier it becomes. With intermittent fasting, your mindset toward eating becomes more purposeful as you focus on your eating-versus-fasting windows. For a lot of people, intermittent fasting becomes so easy and natural to maintain that they begin wondering why they hadn't eaten this way all along.

Keep in mind that *fasting* is a broad term and can mean not eating for days (water fast), skipping one meal a day, or even just eating nothing but soup. As far as intermittent fasting goes, there are many different options, with their own protocols, pros, and cons. All the intermittent fasting methods lead to weight loss and improved health. The one I recommend for its effectiveness and ease of adhering to is the 16:8 method. Going forward, when I refer to *intermittent fasting*, I always mean the 16:8 method.

The Science of Intermittent Fasting

Although fasting has been around for centuries, we are just beginning to fully understand what happens to our bodies when we fast and how doing so affects our health. The first thing your body does when you are not eating is change your hormone levels so that it can continue to get fuel for energy. After about twelve hours of fasting (no eating), the glucose from the food you ate is depleted. As your glucose levels continue to drop, your pancreas no longer needs to produce insulin to keep your blood sugar level under control.

Intermittent fasting can help you live longer. Studies have shown that just by restricting the number of calories you consume every day, you will lengthen your life span. Intermittent fasting is easy once you realize that you don't have to pay so much attention to food in order to lose weight. It's a routine that you can easily adapt to and have great success with.

When your insulin levels are lower, your stored body fat becomes readily available to be used as fuel. Once your body is no longer able to find glucose, it must resort to the glycogen stores in your liver and muscles. Once the glycogen has been consumed, it then turns to stored body fat. Once this happens, the fatty acids produce ketones to provide energy for both your brain and body.

Also, while your insulin levels are lowering, human growth hormone (HGH) levels will increase. Increasing your HGH levels helps to burn stored fat as well as prevent muscle loss in the body. Some studies have shown how fasting for twelve hours can increase your growth hormones by 30 percent, whereas fasting for sixteen hours can give a rise of 200 percent.

When in the fasting state, your cells will start repairing, and this is known as *autophagy*. Autophagy is the body's way of cleaning out damaged cells in order to regenerate newer, healthier cells. Autophagy detoxifies the body and slows the aging process. Autophagy can rev up as early as twelve hours into a fast. This will target the cells that may be full of toxins, bacteria, viruses, and other debris, and it clears them out of the body. So fasting is a great way to detox the body and repair cellular damage.

Common Myths About Intermittent Fasting

There are a lot of misconceptions about intermittent fasting. Here are the most common myths:

Myth 1: You will lose muscle mass.

You may have heard that once you go into starvation mode, you'll lose muscle mass, but studies show that this is not true when intermittent fasting is done correctly. With the increase in growth hormones triggered by intermittent fasting, as shown in some studies, the chances of losing muscle mass are reduced. In fact, your metabolic rate actually increases during short periods of fasting. Your body starts using stored fat for fuel when you aren't eating. The key here is to do intermittent fasting the proper way. Even if you decided to go through long periods of fasting (for several days), eating a high-protein meal just before you begin would supply you with a sufficient amount of amino acids in your bloodstream to prevent muscle degradation. So, you can get rid of the fear of losing muscle mass while intermittent fasting and focus instead on creating your best body.

Myth 2: To lose weight, you must eat five to six small meals a day.

The fact is that your body does need some energy to digest food. You burn about 10 percent of your calories just digesting food. However, studies show that how often one eats has no impact on overall calorie burn during the day, so eating more meals throughout the day will not enhance calorie burn. Some also think that eating protein five to six times per day will support the development of muscles, but studies show that the total amount of protein in a day—not protein every few hours—is what is needed to build and maintain muscle mass. What frequent meals most likely do is help you avoid hunger pangs, which can be managed through self-control and discipline.

Myth 3: Intermittent fasting will cause you to gain weight.

The thought is that you'll be so hungry from fasting that you'll overeat during the eating window. However, this depends on the individual, and most people do not try to overcompensate for the meals missed while fasting. Once your body adjusts to fasting on a daily basis, you will maintain a normal diet during your eight-hour eating window.

Myth 4: You are starving yourself.

You may have heard that intermittent fasting is starving yourself and harmful to your health. Some believe that you are depriving your body of vital nutrients that you need to stay healthy. But understand, there is a difference between starving and simply being hungry. Starvation is when you don't have sufficient food for the body to function. It means you are restricting calories without a choice and there is no food in your future. However, with intermittent fasting, you are purposely choosing to avoid meals and calories for a specified period of time. Then there is a plan to resume eating after that time period. So, it would take several days of not eating at all to have your body go into so-called starvation mode, which does slow down your metabolism. 16:8 intermittent fasting is effectively skipping a meal, and it won't put you in starvation mode or slow your metabolism.

How to Do Intermittent Fasting

Intermittent fasting accelerates the process of getting into ketosis. Quite frankly, nothing lowers insulin faster than eating nothing, and intermittent fasting is a process where you don't eat for long periods of time. Here is a quick summary of the guidelines that will ensure your success while intermittent fasting (16:8).

- Each day you (a) eat healthy meals during the eight-hour window and (b) fast during the sixteen-hour window. Keep in mind, though, that the majority of the sixteen-hour fast happens while you are sleeping. An example would be that you eat no foods after 8 p.m., then you skip breakfast and resume eating after noon the next day. This is an example of a 16:8 hour fast. Another example would be to eat between 10 a.m. and 6 p.m., which allows plenty of time for a healthy breakfast and lunch around midday and a light dinner or snack around 5 or 5:30 p.m., before starting your fast. To avoid disrupting your hormones, it's important to maintain a consistent schedule of fasting and eating times. So, pick a schedule and try to stick with it daily.

- To maximize results, during your eight-hour eating window, you should eat clean and healthy meals, focusing on moderate-protein, low-carb foods and high amounts of healthy fats.

- While fasting, you should drink plenty of fluids. Pure water is most ideal, but you can also have black coffee, green tea, herbal teas, and other no-calorie beverages. Water with lemon, apple cider vinegar, or stevia are also fine, as well as any sugar-free carbonated waters. Staying hydrated will also keep the hunger pangs away.

- You have flexibility during your eight-hour eating window. You could eat two or three meals as long as you keep all eating within the eight-hour window.

- As far as working out, you would think that the sixteen-hour window may not be the most ideal time to work out because many prefer having food or a protein shake just prior to working out. However, if you're able to, you can work out a few hours before breaking your fast. Doing so will allow more growth hormones to be released while your insulin levels are low.

You can measure your level of ketosis through over-the-counter urine tests (keto sticks). Don't, however, become fixated on the results. Pay attention to whether you're losing more fat, feeling more energy, and enjoying better mental clarity, all positive signs that you are in ketosis. I have seen folks get disappointed by the results on the keto stick when their scale clearly indicated they were losing weight. Don't fall for that trap. Focus on the results you're getting.

Tabata

What Is Tabata?

Tabata, also nicknamed the 4-Minute Fat-Burning Miracle, can help you burn more fat than a traditional sixty-minute aerobic workout. Tabata is a type of high-intensity interval training (HIIT) workout invented by Dr. Izumi Tabata, a Japanese physician and researcher. However, Tabata takes HIIT a step further. The intervals are shorter and more intense than most people are used to. Tabata consists of eight intervals, totaling four minutes. Each interval lasts twenty seconds and is followed by ten seconds of rest. Although any type of exercise can be used during Tabata, the key is that it is performed at an absolute maximum intensity for the entirety of the eight intervals.

Studies have confirmed that Tabata can improve cardiovascular health and boost your metabolism and endurance. Tabata will also increase your resting metabolic rate, which will help you burn fat all day long. Tabata can increase both your aerobic and anaerobic capacity, which increases the amount of oxygen used during exercising. This will lead to a healthier heart and lungs.

How to Do Tabata

Do each exercise for twenty seconds followed by a ten-second rest. Complete eight rounds for a total of four minutes. Most people use a free Tabata app as their timer. If you're new to exercising, be sure you do a quick warm-up and stretch before you begin, because Tabata is incredibly intense.

Choose from the following exercises, mixing and matching moves from the list below. Be sure to keep your intensity level high and push yourself as hard as possible during the twenty seconds. You can choose any of the exercises below and find videos on YouTube that will help you learn how to do them:

- Burpees
- Jumping jacks
- Squat jumps
- Speed skaters
- High knees
- Jumping rope
- Mountain climbers
- Suicide runs
- Box jumps
- Butt kicks

Many *really* fall in love with Tabata. It is great for those with a busy schedule. If you're bored with your current work-outs or only have a few minutes, you should give Tabata a try. It will give you results with only a few minutes per day, but beware: it will also wipe you out!

CHAPTER 3

Getting Prepared/What to Expect on the 14-Day New Keto Cleanse

The 14-Day New Keto Cleanse is a health-transforming experience. It will challenge you spiritually, mentally, and physically. It will enhance your life in many positive ways. You will have more control and discipline over your eating habits. You will also learn to have a better relationship with food.

During this 14-Day New Keto Cleanse, there will be times when you feel frustrated or like giving up. But if you stick with it, your body will reward you for your efforts. You will be truly amazed at the results you achieve in just fourteen days!

The first few days—as your body adjusts to the transition to ketosis—will be the most challenging. But this is normal. Later in this chapter, I tell you what common side effects to expect and how to minimize them during the cleanse. After the first few days, your body will become satisfied, with less cravings, and you will begin to feel energized and healthy, maybe for the first time in years.

What to Expect

With the 14-Day New Keto Cleanse, you will

- drop pounds and inches rapidly, losing up to fifteen pounds in two weeks;

- learn how to get your body into ketosis (fat-burning mode) to burn fat faster and more effortlessly;
- learn a four-minute exercise that can speed up fat loss, particularly stubborn body fat;
- shed stubborn fat around your waist, stomach, hips, and thighs that seems impossible to shake;
- lose weight without starving yourself or spending hours in the gym;
- wake up with more energy, clearer thinking, and productive days; and
- slow down the aging process and reverse many health conditions.

Precautions Before Starting the 14-Day New Keto Cleanse

There are certain individuals for whom this program is not ideal:

- people above the age of seventy, unless they are in extremely good health;
- pregnant women;
- people suffering from any disease of the liver or kidneys;
- underweight people and anyone suffering from anorexia; and
- athletes during competition or intense training sessions.

You should get your doctor's approval before you start if you are

- taking insulin or meds that lower blood sugar levels;
- suffering from any disease of the liver or kidneys;

- suffering from hypertension; cancer; or a cardiovascular, neurodegenerative, or autoimmune disease; or
- taking any meds or blood thinners prescribed by your doctor.

Common Side Effects When Starting the 14-Day New Keto Cleanse

There are a few side effects when beginning this program as your body makes the transition to ketosis. You may even have heard these side effects called the *keto flu*. The important thing to remember is that these side effects are temporary and should pass as you enter ketosis.

Headaches

Headaches may occur as the brain is adapting to not having glucose as fuel and switching over to using ketones. Typically, these can last a few days. You can certainly take a painkiller for your headaches and add more sea salt to your diet to minimize them.

Hunger/Cravings

You will feel hungry as you begin this plan and will crave foods that you're used to eating. The cravings will go away within three days, and your body will feel less hungry and more satisfied as you continue the program.

Fatigue/Brain Fog

When your body is adjusting to ketosis, fatigue and brain fog can set in for a few days. This is when you feel tired, disoriented, and distracted. You have a difficult time focusing and concentrating. You feel the need to rest and lie down. Supplementing with B vitamins will give a lot of extra support to make the transition to ketosis easier.

Keto Breath

Those pursuing a keto diet often have fruity-smelling breath, or in some cases, bad breath. This is likely due to acetone, which is a certain type of ketone found in your saliva. Simply by chewing gum or eating mints, you can eliminate this temporary problem.

Gut Issues

This plan limits dietary fiber from fruit, which may affect your normal bowel habits, causing you to feel constipated. To stay regular, increase fiber intake by eating plenty of greens and salads. If you get diarrhea, this could be due to the MCT oil, because too much of it can act as a laxative. If this occurs, you can reduce your consumption of MCT oil, and then gradually increase to a comfortable level.

Sleep Issues

Eliminating carbs may cause insomnia, which is very common. If you struggle with sleep, try to avoid caffeine in the evening and night. If you still struggle with sleeping, you could also try an over-the-counter sleep aid, such as melatonin.

Muscle or Calf Cramps

This is generally caused by an electrolyte deficiency, typically either potassium or magnesium. If this occurs, increase your sea salt intake, because when you're in a low-insulin state, it signals the kidneys to create more sodium, so supplementing with more sea salt helps. You could also take an electrolyte supplement that consists of potassium, magnesium, chloride, calcium, and sodium, and this should solve this problem.

Nausea/Right Shoulder Pain

These issues are generally related to a sluggish gallbladder. When you consume too much fat, nuts, and seeds, you can irritate the gallbladder and its ducts. Nausea or pain can happen because there is not enough bile to handle the extra fat in your diet. Just reduce the amount of fat and gradually increase to higher levels as your body adjusts.

General Guidelines to Minimize and Avoid Common Side Effects

Drink plenty of water.

Throughout this program you should plan on drinking much more water than you typically do. This is because carbs tend to cause your body to hold on to water, so when you reduce the amount of carbs, your body will begin to release the extra water. You will need to replace this water. You may even experience dry mouth when you begin this program. A general guideline is to try to get at least half your body weight in ounces of water daily. For example, if you weigh 180 pounds, you should drink at least ninety ounces of water per day. If you follow a detox program, you may need up to a gallon per day. One habit to maintain is to drink a glass of water when you wake up to hydrate your body from overnight and to set the tone for more water to come throughout the day. You can also slowly drink a glass of water or some coffee once you start feeling hungry. Often, by the time you've finished your drink, your hunger will have passed.

Learn to manage your electrolytes.

Beginning this program and reducing carbs puts your body into a detox period as it flushes excess sugar out of your system. As you go through this adjustment, electrolytes help minimize symptoms such as headaches, cramping, and fatigue. Again, this adjustment period happens only for the first few days on the program.

Gradually increase your fat intake.

It may seem difficult to get enough healthy fats to meet the daily requirements to feel full and satiated. However, adding healthy oils to almost everything you eat helps a lot and allows you to gradually add in more healthy fats.

Get plenty of sea salt.

You don't have to fear salt on this plan because most of the healthy, whole foods you'll be eating don't have much salt in them. My favorite is pink Himalayan salt because it has more minerals than traditional table salt.

Plan ahead before eating out.

The good news is that many restaurants will provide keto-friendly meals if you just ask for them. On the menu, they may also be called *skinny meals* or *low carb* meals. Before you go to a restaurant, you can review the menu online and iden-tify great keto-friendly meals that will comply with this program. Of course, meat or fish are usually a great place to start your meal, and then add green veggies or salads. Be careful of the hidden carbs in sauces and dressings. Ask for those to be left off or placed on the side. You can also replace them with a keto-friendly sauce or dip, such as Tabasco sauce or spinach-artichoke dip.

Leverage supplements that make the program easier and more effective.

In a later chapter, I detail the supplements that allow you to have greater success and fewer side effects during this program. These supplements ease side effects, so you'll be less likely to quit. They also help the body get and stay in fat-burning mode, which is ketosis, the ultimate goal.

Take Measurements

One important reminder before you begin is to weigh yourself, take your measurements (bust, waist, and hips), and record these numbers along with the date. Some people will lose more weight, whereas others will lose more inches, so you want to measure both! On this cleanse, the majority (80 percent) of those following this plan will lose up to fifteen pounds in fourteen days.

Now it's time to take out your tape measure and take your measurements as follows:

Bust: Take it around your back and under your arms. It should wrap around the fullest part of your bust.
Waistline: Measure around the narrowest part of your waist.
Butt/Hips: Place the tape measure at the widest part of your

hips and wrap it around your butt. Measure your results so you can track the inches melting away.

- Weight_____
- Current Bust size (in inches): _____
- Current Waistline (in inches): _____
- Current Butt/Hip (in inches): _____

Next, take photos of your entire body and of your face, close-up. This will enable you to see the physical changes that take place. Many times, you will see a big difference in the whites of your eyes, along with reduced dark circles and puffiness. This way, you can monitor your progress not just by the weight on the scale but by how you look and feel overall.

This isn't just about weight loss, it's about getting healthy. So, you want to monitor your energy, digestion, moods, mental clarity, and radiance of your skin. Get both the health and weight-loss benefits! Don't let the scale become your enemy. Remember, weight loss can move up and down during a cleanse. But in the end, you will lose weight and feel great.

CHAPTER 4

How to Do the 14-Day New Keto Cleanse

The 14-Day New Keto Cleanse is a health-transforming experience. Here is the summary of the 14-Day New Keto Cleanse regimen:

- **Drink Two Keto Smoothies and Eat One Low-Carb, Fat-Burning Meal Daily:** Each day, drink two keto smoothies and eat one low-carb, fat-burning meal for dinner.
- **Enjoy a Variety of Drinks:** Drink up to a gallon of water per day and drink detox or herbal teas as desired. You can also enjoy one cup of coffee or green tea per day. Caffeinated drinks are fine, but no high-sugar drinks, such as sodas or juices.
- **Enjoy a Snack to Avoid Hunger:** You can enjoy one snack, which may include any veggies, peanut butter, almond butter, nuts, seeds, or any of the snack recipes included in this program. You should have no more than one snack during your eight-hour eating window. The goal is to have a snack that is low in sugar/carbs.
- **Follow an Intermittent Fasting Method Daily:** I recommend the 16:8 method, which focuses on when you eat each day.
- **Do Tabata Daily:** A type of four-minute exercise that can

speed up fat loss, particularly stubborn body fat around the waist, stomach, hips, and thighs.

Week I Meal Plan

For week 1, I recommend you follow the eating plan below to simplify things. Following the plan makes things easier so you don't have to live in the kitchen! However, feel free to use any of the alternative keto smoothie and fat-burning meal recipes provided.

DAY	BREAKFAST	LUNCH	DINNER
I	Vanilla Avocado Keto Smoothie	Vanilla Avocado Keto Smoothie	Turkey and Pumpkin Chili
2	Coconut Almond Keto Smoothie	Coconut Almond Keto Smoothie	Turkey and Pumpkin Chili
3	Strawberry Avocado Keto Smoothie	Strawberry Avocado Keto Smoothie	Baked Coconut Shrimp
4	Berry Vanilla Keto Smoothie	Berry Vanilla Keto Smoothie	Baked Coconut Shrimp
5	Chocolate Keto Smoothie	Chocolate Keto Smoothie	Turkey Sausage Frittata
6	Strawberry Almond Keto Smoothie	Strawberry Almond Keto Smoothie	Turkey Sausage Frittata
7	Peppermint Keto Smoothie	Peppermint Keto Smoothie	Baked Swordfish Packets

Week 2 Meal Plan

For week 2, I recommend you follow the eating plan on the next page to simplify things. However, feel free to use any of the alternative keto smoothie and fat-burning meal recipes provided.

DAY	BREAKFAST	LUNCH	DINNER
8	Vanilla Avocado Keto Smoothie	Vanilla Avocado Keto Smoothie	Baked Swordfish Packets
9	Coconut Almond Keto Smoothie	Coconut Almond Keto Smoothie	Veggie Stir-Fry with Ginger and Cashews
10	Strawberry Avocado Keto Smoothie	Strawberry Avocado Keto Smoothie	Veggie Stir-Fry with Ginger and Cashews
11	Berry Vanilla Keto Smoothie	Berry Vanilla Keto Smoothie	Parmesan Zucchini Noodles with Roasted Tomatoes
12	Chocolate Keto Smoothie	Chocolate Keto Smoothie	Parmesan Zucchini Noodles with Roasted Tomatoes
13	Strawberry Almond Keto Smoothie	Strawberry Almond Keto Smoothie	One Skillet Chicken Fajitas
14	Peppermint Keto Smoothie	Peppermint Keto Smoothie	One Skillet Chicken Fajitas

How to Customize the Plan

If you decide to customize week 1 or 2 of the meal plan, use the blank chart on the next page to write in the keto smoothies and fat-burning meals you plan to eat. Remember that the shopping lists are for the designed plan, so if you customize the plan, you may need to change the shopping lists. The smoothie recipes all yield a single serving, because folks usually prefer to make them fresh, one at a time. The meal recipes are meant to cover more than one day, so they will always yield more than one serving.

DAY	BREAKFAST	LUNCH	DINNER
——	————————	————————	————————
——	————————	————————	————————
——	————————	————————	————————
——	————————	————————	————————
——	————————	————————	————————
——	————————	————————	————————
——	————————	————————	————————

Day 15: Transition Day

A transition day marks the end of the 14-Day New Keto Cleanse and the beginning of a plan you can follow for life. You now have a wider range of meals and smoothies that you can choose each day. Day 15 should feature "soft" meals such as soup, veggies, salads, or green smoothies. Be sure to have complex carbohydrates (vegetables, fruits, etc.) and minimize the consumption of red meat, saturated fats, pastries, cheeses, milk, etc., for the day. The general thought is to eat clean and healthy, avoid processed foods, and focus on veggies, soups, salads, green smoothies, chicken, turkey, fish/seafood, etc.

It's important to remember not to binge on food on day 15. Gradually return to your normal foods over the next twelve hours. The pancreas and liver need to shift back into normal function after a detox cleanse.

Fat Burner Soup

A popular transition meal you can have on day 15 is the Fat Burner Soup. This soup is packed with nutritional powerhouses such as sweet potato, spinach, garlic, carrots, and tomatoes. It flushes the fat away by restoring acid-alkaline and sodium-potassium balance to the body's organs and glands.

The superfoods in this soup contain antioxidants and fiber, which aid in flushing toxins and, subsequently, fat from the body. The soup is warming and deliciously comforting.

Ingredients

I medium sweet potato, peeled and cut into small cubes

3 carrots, peeled and sliced

I stalk celery, diced

I small yellow onion, diced

I teaspoon minced garlic (I clove)

¼ teaspoon of sea salt (more or less to desired taste)

½ teaspoon black pepper

⅛ teaspoon allspice

I teaspoon paprika

I bay leaf

Two 15-ounce cans kidney or navy beans, drained and rinsed

4 cups low-sodium vegetable broth

One 14.5-ounce can diced tomatoes (no salt added)

4 cups baby spinach, loosely packed

I tablespoon extra-virgin olive oil for serving (optional)

Directions

Except for the spinach and olive oil, add all of the ingredients to a slow cooker or large pot. Cover and cook on low to simmer for 6 to 8 hours. Once the vegetables are tender, the soup is ready.

Add the spinach, and continue cooking for 5 to 7 minutes until spinach is wilted.

To make a thicker soup, you can mash some of the vegetables with a fork once they are tender (typically after 5 to 7 hours). Another option to make the soup thicker is to remove I to I½ cups of the soup (liquid only). However, most enjoy it as is, so feel free to serve and enjoy!

Prior to serving, drizzle a little olive oil over the bowl of soup to help enhance the flavor and help the body absorb the nutrients.

After day 15, you can continue intermittent fasting and enjoying the daily regimen of keto smoothies and low-carb, fat-burning meals to continue on your journey.

What to Drink on the 14-Day New Keto Cleanse

The New Keto Cleanse has a lot of flexibility, as the following drinks are recommended:

- Plenty of water (up to a gallon per day)
- Herbal teas
- Bone broth
- One cup of coffee or green tea per day with a splash of dairy or nondairy creamer and stevia/monk fruit

What is not allowed:

- Alcohol
- Sodas, including diet sodas
- Juices
- Coconut water

What Drinks to Enjoy During Your Sixteen-Hour Fasting Window

Many ask, "What can I drink while fasting?" or "What drinks are safe to consume during my sixteen-hour window?" These drinks will not break your fast:

- Plain water
- Water with lemon

- Sparkling mineral water
- Unsweetened tea/coffee (green tea/black tea/herbal teas)
- Apple cider vinegar
- *Not* bone broth (Note: It is *not* allowed during the fasting window but is perfectly fine during your eating window.)

Shopping List for Week I

Here is the shopping list for the first seven days, including both keto smoothies and fat-burning meal recipes. If you choose to use an alternative recipe, be sure to add those ingredients to the shopping list.

- 1 medium yellow or white onion
- 1 medium green bell pepper
- 1 zucchini
- 16 grape tomatoes
- 12 small green pitted olives
- 2 fresh thyme sprigs
- 4 lemons
- 12 eggs
- 1¼ pounds lean ground turkey
- 2 peeled medium garlic cloves, minced
- 8 ounces (about 16) large shrimp
- 6 ounces turkey sausage
- Two 5-ounce skinless swordfish steaks, or any whitefish
- One 14-ounce can reduced-sodium diced tomatoes
- One 15-ounce can pumpkin (do not use pumpkin-pie filling, which is pre-sweetened)

- Unsweetened shredded coconut (sometimes sold as "desiccated")
- Unseasoned whole-wheat or gluten-free panko bread crumbs
- *Sea salt and black pepper
- *Seasonings: chili powder, ground cumin, dried oregano, yellow or red curry powder, red pepper flakes, dried thyme, five-spice powder (Note: Five-spice powder is a traditional Chinese blend, made with cinnamon or acacia and other aromatic spices.)
- *Nonstick cooking spray, aluminum foil, parchment paper
- *Snacks and beverages of your choice: water, teas, coffee, green tea, apples, raw veggies, peanut butter, almond butter, nuts and seeds, etc.
- *1 carton unsweetened vanilla almond milk (½ gallon)
- 1 large container baby spinach (16 ounces)
- 5 medium avocados (or one bag frozen avocado chunks)
- 1 medium banana
- 1 small bag frozen strawberries
- 1 small bag frozen blueberries
- *1 small container MCT oil
- *1 small container coconut oil (not liquid)
- *1 small container almond butter
- *1 package ground flaxseeds
- *1 box stevia packets
- *1 container vanilla plant-based protein powder (e.g., Purely Inspired)
- Four 5.3-ounce cups vanilla yogurt (e.g., Dannon Oikos Triple Zero brand)

- *1 small container cocoa powder (e.g., Hershey's Cocoa Natural Unsweetened)
- *1 small bottle peppermint extract

Note: Items marked with an asterisk can be bought in bulk to last through both weeks.

Shopping List for Week 2

Here is the shopping list for the last seven days, including both keto smoothies and fat-burning meal recipes. If you choose to use an alternative recipe, be sure to add those ingredients to the shopping list. Note that the Fat Burner Soup is optional and not included in this list.

- 10 ounces boneless skinless chicken breast cut for stir-fry, any seasoning packet discarded
- 1 pound frozen vegetables for stir-fry, any flavoring packet discarded
- 1 container grated parmesan cheese
- Minced peeled fresh ginger
- 1 container minced peeled garlic
- 1 small red onion
- 1 small red bell pepper
- 1 small green bell pepper
- 1 small lime
- Cherry tomatoes (for 1 cup)
- 1½ pounds spiralized zucchini (can purchase already spiralized)
- Stemmed fresh thyme leaves

- 1 small container lemon juice
- Natural-style creamy peanut butter
- Bag roasted cashews
- Extra-virgin olive oil
- Low-sodium soy sauce
- Unseasoned rice vinegar (Note: Unseasoned rice vinegar is a low-acid vinegar made without any added sugar.)
- *Sea salt and black pepper
- *Seasonings: chili powder, ground cumin, onion powder, red pepper flakes, dried thyme
- *Nonstick cooking spray
- *Snacks and beverages of your choice: water, teas, coffee, green tea, apples, raw veggies, peanut butter, almond butter, nuts and seeds, etc.
- *1 carton unsweetened vanilla almond milk (½ gallon)
- 1 large container baby spinach (16 ounces)
- 5 medium avocados (or one bag frozen avocado chunks)
- 1 medium banana
- 1 small bag frozen strawberries
- 1 small bag frozen blueberries
- *1 small container MCT oil
- *1 small container coconut oil (not liquid)
- *1 small container almond butter
- *1 package ground flaxseeds
- *1 box stevia packets
- *1 container vanilla plant-based protein powder (e.g., Purely Inspired)
- Four 5.3-ounce cups vanilla yogurt (e.g., Dannon Oikos Triple Zero brand)

- *1 small container cocoa powder (e.g., Hershey's Cocoa Natural Unsweetened)
- *1 small bottle peppermint extract

Weekly Checklist

You can make a copy of this chart below and use it to ensure that all four pillars are completed each day. This will help you stay on track and get the best results.

DAY	2 KETO SMOOTHIES	FAT-BURNING MEAL	INTERMITTENT FASTING (16:8)	TABATA
1	_____	_____	_____	_____
2	_____	_____	_____	_____
3	_____	_____	_____	_____
4	_____	_____	_____	_____
5	_____	_____	_____	_____
6	_____	_____	_____	_____
7	_____	_____	_____	_____

Supportive Supplements

I suggest you purchase these supportive supplements before you start to ensure that your results are maximized and side effects are minimized.

Electrolyte powder (sugar-free)

A mineral/electrolyte supplement will ensure that specific bodily functions run at optimal levels during a detox cleanse. Electrolytes, such as magnesium, potassium, and sodium, play a vital role in the detoxifying/fasting process. Electrolytes support cellular function and help eliminate toxins from the body. I recommend a sugar-free electrolyte powder drink with this program.

Liver Focus

One reason the Liver Focus supplement enhances weight loss is because of the relationship between the liver, mitochondria, and ketones. Ketones are made by mitochondria inside liver cells, so how quickly you make ketones depends on the health of your liver. A healthy liver (i.e., healthy liver cells) will quickly produce ketones. That's why a fatty liver—due not to drinking alcohol but to years of consuming sugar, carbs, and junk food—can make the transition from sugar fuel to fat fuel very difficult. So, be sure to use Liver Focus to improve the health of the liver and help accelerate the body's ability to burn fat. Liver Focus can be found only at www.JJSmithOnline.com.

Blood Sugar Focus

Blood Sugar Focus (BSF) is a supplement that helps to manage healthy blood sugar levels by reducing glucose absorption and glucose production by your body. It also manages the hormone insulin, which is key to helping the body get into ketosis. It also provides specific support for PCOS (polycystic ovary syndrome), pre-diabetes (insulin resistance), and diabetes. BSF not only has both chromium and alpha-lipoic acid (ALA), it features Eriomin, which is patented and clinically proven to reverse insulin resistance. Blood Sugar Focus can be found only at www.JJSmithOnline.com.

MCT oil

A popular ingredient in the keto community is MCT oil. MCT oil is a healthy fat found in foods like coconut oil that is metabolized differently than the long-chain triglycerides (LCT) found in other foods. Since the MCT is digested quicker than the LCT, it gets to be used as energy first, and many find that it improves energy, brain function, and mental clarity. You can even add it to your smoothies and it won't alter the flavor. As you continue on the program and get healthier, you'll need to add MCT oil less often.

CHAPTER 5

The Keto Smoothie Recipes

On the 14-Day New Keto Cleanse, you will detox with keto-friendly smoothies, each designed to be under fifteen net carbs per serving, that are lower in carbs and lower in sugar than traditional green smoothies.

Here are some tips for making keto smoothies:

- **Important:** Please note that many people like to make their smoothies fresh, so my recipes provide one serving. To make two servings at a time, such as for breakfast and lunch, *simply double the recipe*. I also suggest that you highlight which of the first seven keto smoothies you loved so you can remake those during the second week, or use any of the alternative keto smoothie recipes.

- Keto-friendly smoothies are lower in carbs and lower in sugar than traditional green smoothies, so adding a natural sweetener like stevia or monk fruit will be critical for your desired taste.

- With traditional green smoothies, stevia is often not needed due to the amount of fruit in them. However, with keto smoothies, stevia or another natural sweetener (e.g., monk fruit) is often required if it's included in the recipe. So, begin with the amount of stevia in the recipe and then taste it after blending; add more sweetener until you reach your desired sweetness.

- Although avocados have no taste in a smoothie, they are a key ingredient in keto smoothies to ensure they're creamy. You can use frozen avocado chunks, and if you choose to, a half cup of avocado chunks is equal to one half of a medium avocado.

- Certain recipes include protein powder, and of course, you can add protein powder to any of the recipes. The recipes included here were made with plant-based vanilla protein powder, low in sugar. The brand name is Purely Inspired. However, feel free to use any plant-based vanilla protein powder of your choice.

- To make a smoothie colder and less thick, just add more ice to your desired preference.

- Regular, dry measuring cups are fine to use for measuring the ingredients in the keto smoothies.

The Keto Smoothie Recipes

Vanilla Avocado Keto Smoothie

Coconut Almond Keto Smoothie

Strawberry Avocado Keto Smoothie

Berry Vanilla Keto Smoothie

Chocolate Keto Smoothie

Strawberry Almond Keto Smoothie

Peppermint Keto Smoothie

The Alternate Keto Smoothie Recipes

Avocado Butter Keto Smoothie

Banana Lime Keto Smoothie

Blueberry Avocado Keto Smoothie

Almond Butter Banana Keto Smoothie

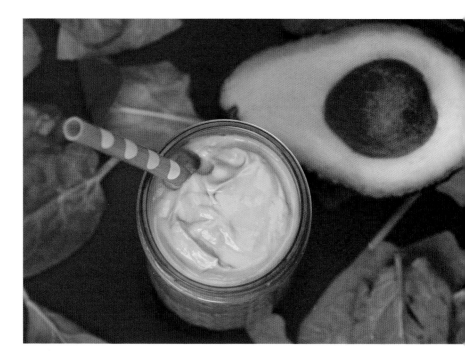

Vanilla Avocado Keto Smoothie

Makes I serving

Ingredients:

¾ cup unsweetened vanilla almond milk

½ cup ice

I cup baby spinach, packed

½ medium avocado, pitted and scooped from shell

I tablespoon MCT oil

I stevia packet (more or less to desired sweetness)

I teaspoon plant-based vanilla protein powder

Directions:

Place all ingredients in the blender and blend until smooth and creamy in consistency.

Coconut Almond Keto Smoothie

Makes 1 serving

Ingredients:

½ cup unsweetened vanilla almond milk

1 cup ice

1 cup baby spinach, packed

½ medium banana

1 tablespoon almond butter

1 tablespoon coconut oil

1 stevia packet (more or less to desired sweetness)

Directions:

Place all ingredients in the blender and blend until smooth and creamy in consistency.

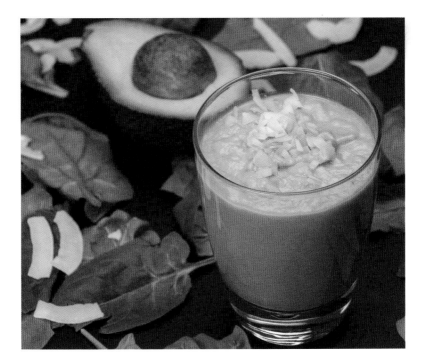

Strawberry Avocado Keto Smoothie

Makes 1 serving

Ingredients:

3/4 cup unsweetened vanilla almond milk

1/2 cup ice

2 cups baby spinach, packed

1/2 cup frozen strawberries

1/2 medium avocado, pitted and scooped from shell

2 tablespoons ground flaxseeds

2 stevia packets (more or less to desired sweetness)

Directions:

Place all ingredients in the blender and blend until smooth and creamy in consistency.

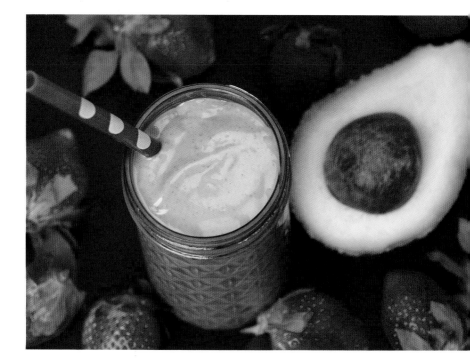

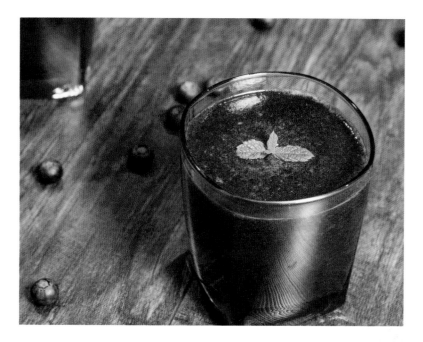

Berry Vanilla Keto Smoothie
Makes I serving

Ingredients:
¼ cup water

2 cups baby spinach, packed

½ cup frozen blueberries

One 5.3-ounce cup vanilla yogurt (e.g., Dannon Oikos Triple Zero
  brand)

I tablespoon MCT oil

I stevia packet (more or less to desired sweetness)

Directions:
Place all ingredients in the blender and blend until smooth and creamy
in consistency.

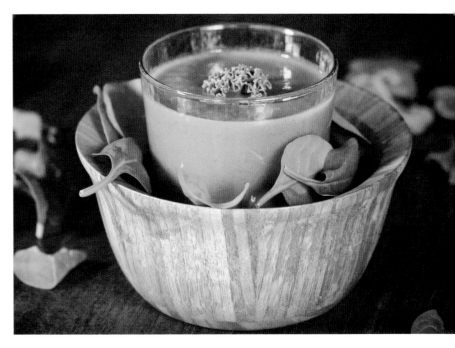

Chocolate Keto Smoothie

Makes I serving

Ingredients:

1/2 cup unsweetened vanilla almond milk

1/2 cup ice

I cup baby spinach, packed

1/2 medium avocado, pitted and scooped from shell

One 5.3-ounce cup vanilla yogurt (e.g., Dannon Oikos Triple Zero brand)

I teaspoon cocoa powder (e.g., Hershey's Cocoa Natural Unsweetened)

I tablespoon MCT oil

2 stevia packets (more or less to desired sweetness)

Directions:

Place all ingredients in the blender and blend until smooth and creamy in consistency.

Strawberry Almond Keto Smoothie

Makes 1 serving

Ingredients:

½ cup unsweetened vanilla almond milk

½ cup ice

2 cups baby spinach, packed

¼ cup frozen strawberries

½ medium avocado, pitted and scooped from shell

1 tablespoon coconut oil

1 stevia packet (more or less to desired sweetness)

2 teaspoons plant-based vanilla protein powder

Directions:

Place all ingredients in the blender and blend until smooth and creamy in consistency.

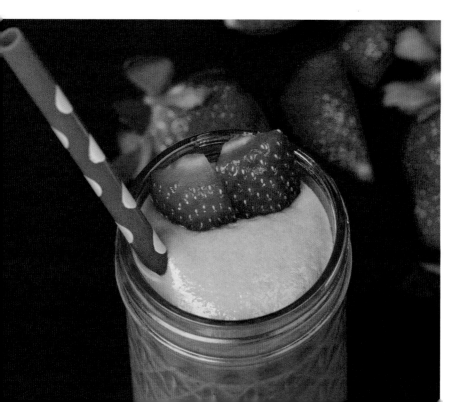

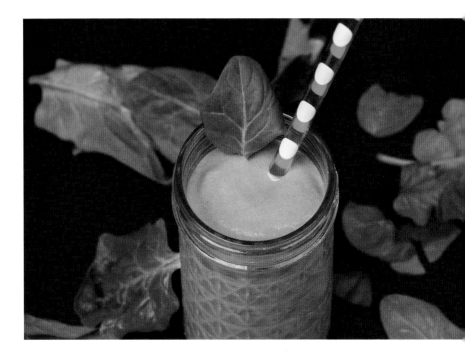

Peppermint Keto Smoothie

Makes I serving

Ingredients:

3⁄4 cup unsweetened vanilla almond milk

I cup ice

I cup baby spinach, packed

1⁄2 medium avocado, pitted and scooped from shell

I tablespoon ground flaxseeds

1⁄4 teaspoon peppermint extract or I handful fresh mint leaves

I1⁄2 stevia packets (more or less to desired sweetness)

2 teaspoons plant-based vanilla protein powder

Directions:

Place all ingredients in the blender and blend until smooth and creamy in consistency.

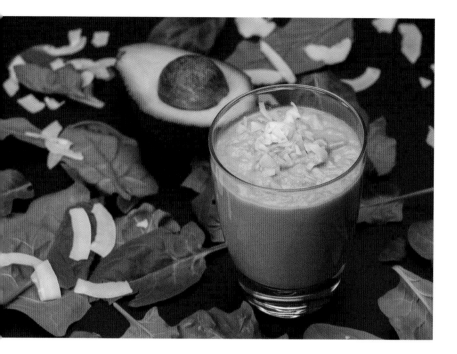

Avocado Butter Keto Smoothie

Makes 1 serving

Ingredients:

3/4 cup unsweetened vanilla almond milk

1/2 cup ice

1 cup baby spinach, packed

1/2 medium avocado, pitted and scooped from shell

1 tablespoon almond butter

1 stevia packet (more or less to desired sweetness)

2 teaspoons plant-based vanilla protein powder

Directions:

Place all ingredients in the blender and blend until smooth and creamy in consistency.

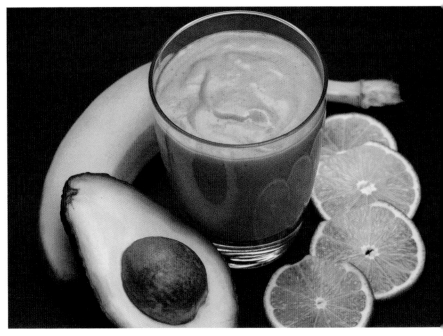

Banana Lime Keto Smoothie

Makes 1 serving

Ingredients:

¾ cup unsweetened vanilla almond milk

1 cup ice

1 cup baby spinach, packed

¼ medium banana

1 medium avocado, pitted and scooped from shell

2 tablespoons lime juice

½ teaspoon cinnamon

1 stevia packet (more or less to desired sweetness)

2 teaspoons plant-based vanilla protein powder

Directions:

Place all ingredients in the blender and blend until smooth and creamy in consistency.

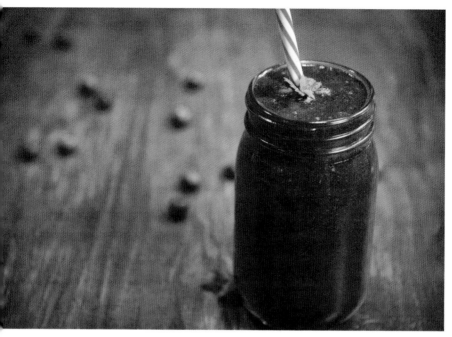

Blueberry Avocado Keto Smoothie

Makes 1 serving

Ingredients:

3/4 cup unsweetened vanilla almond milk

1/2 cup ice

2 cups baby spinach, packed

1/2 medium avocado, pitted and scooped from shell

1/2 cup frozen blueberries

2 tablespoons ground flaxseeds

2 stevia packets (more or less to desired sweetness)

Directions:

Place all ingredients in the blender and blend until smooth and creamy in consistency.

Almond Butter Banana Keto Smoothie

Makes 1 serving

Ingredients:

½ cup unsweetened vanilla almond milk

½ cup ice

1 cup baby spinach, packed

½ medium banana

1½ tablespoons almond butter

1 stevia packet (more or less to desired sweetness)

Directions:

Place all ingredients in the blender and blend until smooth and creamy in consistency.

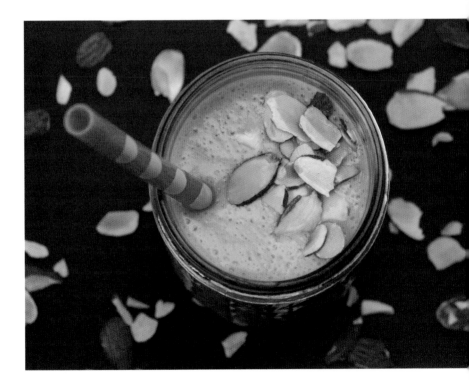

CHAPTER 6

The Low Carb, Fat-Burning Meals and Snack Recipes

Everything—from what you eat to what you drink to when you consume it—affects your weight. That is why it is important to eat foods that not only taste good but also help to shed fat.

The 14-Day New Keto Cleanse includes hot meals that are low carb and low sugar, with moderate protein and healthy fats to ensure maximum fat loss. This cleanse provides a more balanced approach to eating good carbs, healthy fats, and lean protein that prevents rebound weight gain.

This plan includes forty new recipes (eleven keto smoothies and twenty-nine meal and snack recipes). Eating these fat-burning meals can help you

- burn fat faster,
- rev up your metabolism,
- feel fuller longer, and
- build muscle that naturally burns more calories than fat.

When a person adds these fat-burning meals to their diet, they can burn fat and lose weight over time. The term *fat-burning meal* applies to those meals designed to promote fat loss by revving up the metabolism, reducing appetite, and reducing the overall sugar/carb intake.

You will enjoy this healthy eating plan that will help you balance hormones, decrease hunger, regulate your metabolism, and remove toxins that lead to chronic disease. The foods in the fat-burning meal recipes include lean proteins, good carbs, and healthy fats at each meal.

The Low-Carb, Fat-Burning Meal Recipes

Turkey and Pumpkin Chili (4 servings)

Baked Coconut Shrimp (2 servings)

Turkey Sausage Frittata (4 servings)

Baked Swordfish Packets (2 servings)

Veggie Stir-Fry with Ginger and Cashews (2 Servings)

Parmesan Zucchini Noodles with
Roasted Tomatoes (4 servings)

One-Skillet Chicken Fajitas (2 servings)

The Alternate Low-Carb,
Fat-Burning Meal Recipes

Chicken Lettuce Wraps (2 servings)

Oven-Roasted Sausage and Peppers (2 servings)

Pork and Pineapple Kebabs with Fresh Salsa (4 servings)

Enlightened Egg Salad (3 servings)

Oven-Fried Cod Cakes (2 servings)

Warm Tuna with Roasted Cauliflower
and Olives (2 servings)

Apple-Almond Meatballs in an Herbed
Tomato Sauce (4 servings)

Sheet-Pan Salmon (2 servings)

Warm Kale Salad with Chicken, Pine Nuts,
and Tomatoes (2 servings)

Herb Pesto Baked Shrimp (4 servings)

Spinach and Scallion Mini Muffins (2 servings)

Shrimp Egg Roll Salad (1 serving)

The Snack Recipes

Super Simple Parmesan Pizza Chips

Crispy Curried Chickpeas

Spicy Asparagus Spears with Turkey Bacon

Cucumber Tomato Salad

White Bean Hummus

Tomato Avocado Salad

Air-Fried Avocado

Tuna Avocado Boats

Deviled Avocado Eggs

Cauliflower Flatbread

Turkey and Pumpkin Chili

Makes 4 servings

Ingredients:

Nonstick cooking spray

1 medium yellow or white onion, chopped (1 cup)

1 medium green bell pepper, stemmed, cored, and chopped (1 cup)

1¼ pounds lean ground turkey

3 tablespoons chili powder, or to taste

2 teaspoons ground cumin

1 teaspoon dried oregano

1 teaspoon table salt

One 14-ounce can reduced-sodium diced tomatoes

¾ cup canned pumpkin (do not use pumpkin-pie filling, which is pre-
    sweetened)

½ cup water

Directions:

Spray the inside of a medium Dutch oven or a large saucepan with
nonstick cooking spray and warm over medium heat. Add the onion
and bell pepper; cook for 3 minutes, stirring occasionally, or until the
onion softens.

Crumble in the ground turkey. Cook for 2 minutes, stirring often, or
until lightly browned.

Stir in the chili powder, cumin, oregano, and salt until uniform.
Then stir in the diced tomatoes, pumpkin, and water until uniform.
Bring to a simmer, stirring frequently.

Cover, reduce the heat to very low, and simmer slowly, stirring
occasionally until thickened a bit, about 20 minutes. Serve hot.

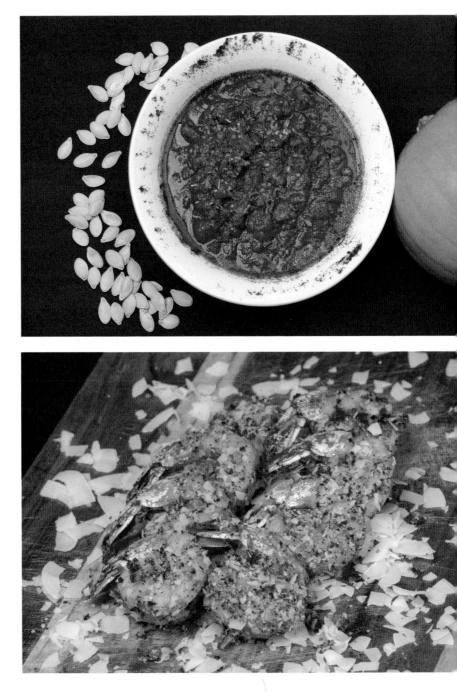

Baked Coconut Shrimp

Makes 2 servings

Ingredients:

¼ cup unsweetened shredded coconut (sometimes sold as "desiccated")

½ cup unseasoned whole-wheat or gluten-free panko bread crumbs

½ teaspoon yellow or red curry powder

¼ teaspoon table salt

I large egg white

8 ounces (or I6) large shrimp, peeled and deveined

Nonstick cooking spray

Directions:

Position the rack in the oven's center and heat the oven to 375°F.

Pulse the coconut, bread crumbs, curry powder, and salt in a food processor two or three times until lightly ground. Pour this mixture into a medium bowl.

Whisk the egg white in a second medium bowl until foamy.

Pour the shrimp into the egg white and toss well to coat evenly and thoroughly.

Coat a lipped baking sheet with nonstick cooking spray. Use your cleaned hands to dip the coated shrimp one at a time into the coconut mixture. Transfer them to the baking sheet as you work, spacing them a couple of inches apart. Lightly spray the top of the shrimp with the nonstick spray.

Bake for I5 minutes, or until crisp and lightly browned. Cool for 5 minutes but serve warm.

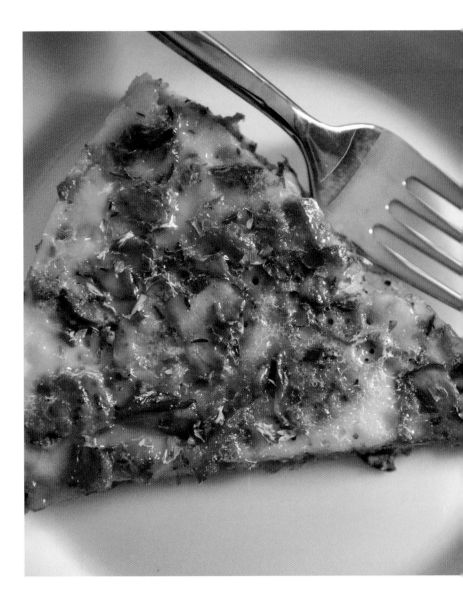

Turkey Sausage Frittata

Makes 4 servings

Ingredients:

6 ounces turkey sausage, any casings removed
2 peeled medium garlic cloves, minced (about 2 teaspoons)
1/2 teaspoon dried thyme
Up to 1/2 teaspoon red pepper flakes
1/2 teaspoon salt
6 large eggs, whisked until smooth

Directions:

Warm a 10-inch nonstick skillet over medium heat. Crumble in the turkey sausage and cook for 6 to 8 minutes, stirring frequently, or until the meat browns a little.

Stir in the garlic, thyme, red pepper flakes, and salt. Then reduce the heat to low and pour the whisked eggs all around the skillet, not just in its center. Cover and cook for 10 minutes, until the top of the frittata is set and does not jiggle when you shake the pan.

Use a spatula to loosen the frittata from the edges and bottom of the pan. Slip it onto a cutting board. Cut into quarters to serve.

Baked Swordfish Packets

Makes 2 servings

Ingredients:

Two 5-ounce skinless swordfish steaks

1 cup diced zucchini

16 grape tomatoes, halved

12 small green pitted olives, thinly sliced

2 fresh thyme sprigs

4 lemon wedges

1/2 teaspoon table salt

1/2 teaspoon ground black pepper

Directions:

Position the rack in the oven's center and heat the oven to 400°F.

Lay one 16-inch piece of aluminum foil on your work surface so that one long side faces you. Cover it with one sheet of 16-inch parchment paper.

Set one fish in the center of the parchment paper. Scatter half the zucchini, tomatoes, and olives over the fish and in a line parallel to the long side of the parchment paper, leaving at least a 2-inch border on each end. Lay a thyme sprig on the fish, then squeeze 2 lemon wedges over everything (catch the seeds!) and drop the wedges among the vegetables. Sprinkle everything with half of the salt and pepper.

Bring the long ends of the parchment and foil together and crimp them into a tight seal, using the foil to catch and hold the parchment paper. Roll the short ends up, creating a tight seal on each end. Transfer the packet to a baking sheet.

Repeat for the second swordfish.

Bake for 20 minutes. Transfer the baking sheet to a wire rack and cool for 5 minutes before opening. Remove from parchment paper before serving.

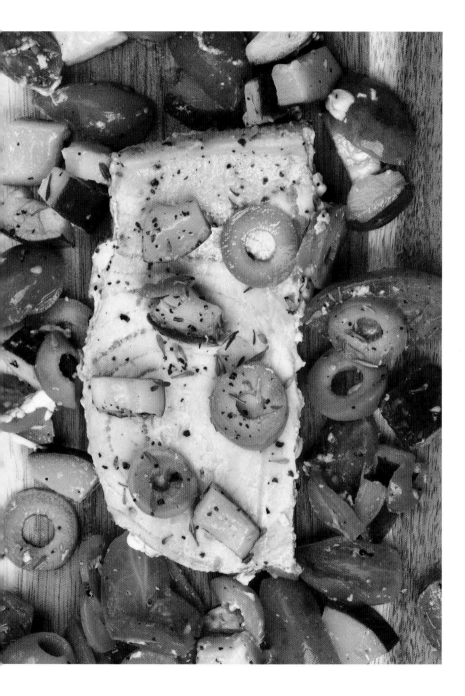

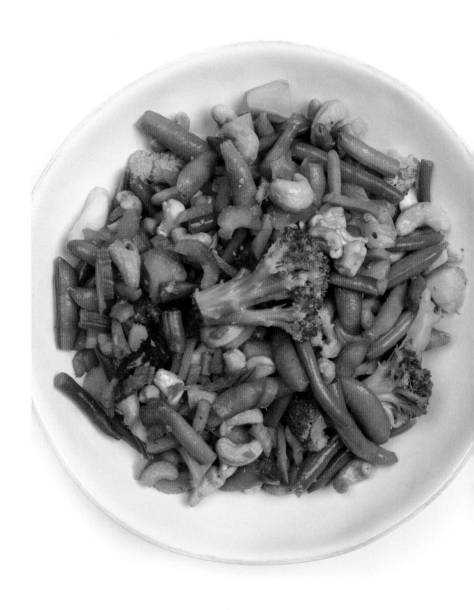

Veggie Stir-Fry with Ginger and Cashews

Makes 2 servings

Ingredients:

2 tablespoons low-sodium soy sauce

I tablespoon unseasoned rice vinegar

I tablespoon natural-style creamy peanut butter

I pound frozen vegetables for stir-fry, any flavoring
   packet discarded

Nonstick cooking spray

I tablespoon minced peeled fresh ginger

2 teaspoons minced peeled garlic

¼ cup roasted cashews

Directions:

Whisk the soy sauce, vinegar, and peanut butter in a small bowl until smooth. Set aside.

Use your cleaned hands to gently squeeze the thawed vegetables in small batches over the sink to remove excess moisture. Don't crush the vegetables. Set them aside.

Coat the inside of a large nonstick skillet or wok with nonstick cooking spray. Warm over medium-high heat, then add the ginger and garlic. Stir-fry for 30 seconds, or until fragrant.

Add the vegetables and continue stir-frying for 2 minutes, or until heated through. Add the cashews and toss well.

Pour in the soy sauce mixture and stir-fry for I minute, until the sauce is a bit thickened and the vegetables are coated. Serve hot.

Parmesan Zucchini Noodles with Roasted Tomatoes

Makes 4 servings

Ingredients:

1 cup cherry tomatoes, cut in half

4 tablespoons olive oil

1/2 teaspoon salt

1/2 teaspoon ground black pepper

1 1/2 pounds spiralized zucchini

1 1/2 tablespoons lemon juice

2 teaspoons stemmed fresh thyme leaves

1/2 cup finely grated Parmesan cheese

Directions:

Preheat the oven to 400°F. Distribute the cherry tomatoes evenly on a baking sheet. Drizzle with 2 tablespoons of olive oil and season with half of the salt and pepper. Transfer the baking sheet into the oven and roast for 10 to 15 minutes until the cherry tomatoes just start to burst. Remove the baking sheet and set aside.

Add 2 tablespoons oil to a large skillet, swirl it around to coat the bottom, then add the zucchini noodles. Cook, stirring constantly, for 2 minutes, until just wilted.

Add the lemon juice, thyme, and remaining salt and pepper. Stir well. Then add the cherry tomatoes and the cheese. Toss lightly until well combined. Serve warm.

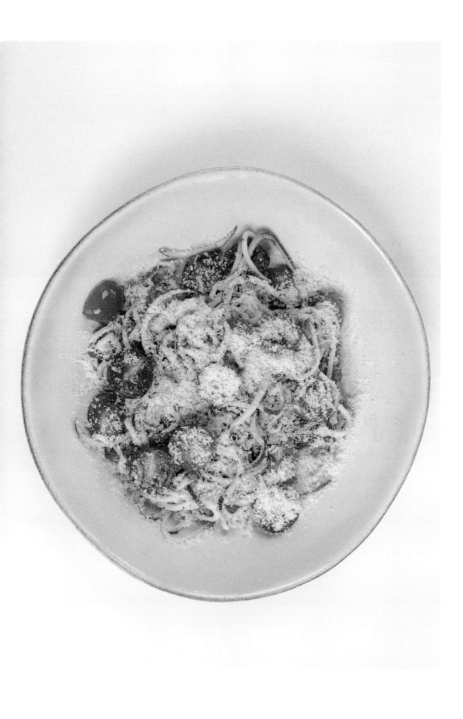

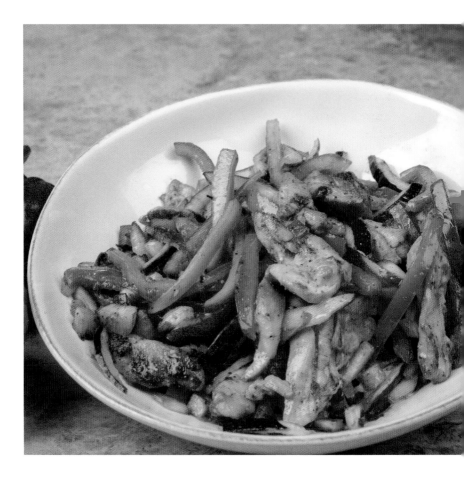

One-Skillet Chicken Fajitas

Makes 2 servings

Ingredients:

10 ounces boneless skinless chicken breast cut for stir-fry, any
    seasoning packet discarded

2 teaspoons regular chili powder

1/2 teaspoon ground cumin

1/2 teaspoon onion powder

1/4 teaspoon table salt

2 teaspoons olive oil

1 small red onion, thinly sliced

1 small red bell pepper, stemmed, cored, and thinly sliced

1 small green bell pepper, stemmed, cored, and thinly sliced

1 1/2 teaspoons minced garlic (1 large peeled clove)

1 small lime, halved

Directions:

Stir the chicken, chili powder, cumin, onion powder, and salt in a
medium bowl until the meat is evenly coated in the spices.

Warm 1 teaspoon oil in a medium nonstick skillet set over medium-
high heat. Add the chicken and all spices in the bowl. Cook for
4 minutes, stirring and tossing often, or until lightly browned.

Transfer the chicken to a plate. Add the remaining 1 teaspoon oil to
the skillet; add the onion, bell peppers, and garlic. Cook for 3 minutes,
stirring often, or until the onions soften and the bell peppers just start
to blister.

Return the chicken and any juices to the skillet. Stir well to warm
through. Remove the skillet from the heat and squeeze the lime over
the chicken mixture. Stir well and enjoy warm.

Chicken Lettuce Wraps

Makes 2 servings

Ingredients:

Two 5-ounce boneless skinless chicken breasts

1 teaspoon toasted sesame oil

1/4 teaspoon five-spice powder or ground cinnamon

Nonstick cooking spray

1/2 medium red bell pepper, cored and julienned

1 medium carrot, shredded

1/2 cup bean sprouts

1 1/2 tablespoons low-sodium soy sauce

1 tablespoon unseasoned rice vinegar

2 teaspoons Worcestershire sauce

1 teaspoon bottled ginger juice

6 Boston lettuce leaves

Directions:

Rub the chicken breasts with the sesame oil and sprinkle them with the five-spice powder or cinnamon.

Lightly coat the inside of a medium nonstick skillet with nonstick cooking spray. Warm it over medium heat, then add the chicken breasts. Cook for 8 minutes, turning once, or until cooked through. Transfer the chicken breasts to a cutting board and cool for 5 minutes before slicing them into thin strips.

Toss the bell pepper, carrot, bean sprouts, soy sauce, vinegar, Worcestershire sauce, and ginger juice in a medium bowl until the vegetables are well coated. Add the chicken and toss well.

Lay 3 lettuce leaves on each of two plates. Top each leaf with about 2/3 cup of the chicken mixture. Roll up the leaves like wraps to enjoy them!

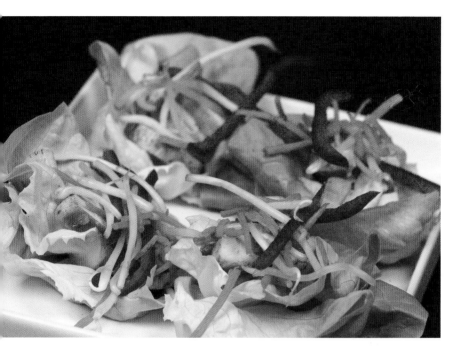

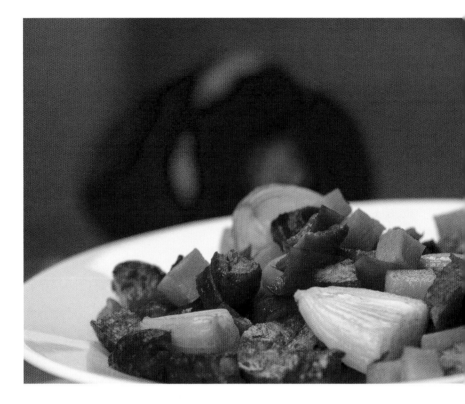

Oven-Roasted Sausage and Peppers

Makes 2 servings

Ingredients:

8 ounces Italian-style turkey or chicken sausage, cut into 1½-inch
    pieces

I medium red bell pepper, stemmed, cored, and cut into 1½-inch pieces

8 ounces peeled, seeded, and cubed butternut squash (½-inch
    pieces)

2 large shallots, peeled and quartered

Olive oil spray

I tablespoon balsamic vinegar or white balsamic vinegar

Directions:

Position the rack in the oven's center and heat the oven to 375°F.

Put the sausage pieces, bell pepper, squash, and shallots in a
9-x-13-inch baking pan. Spray generously with olive oil spray and toss
to coat well.

Bake for 45 minutes, tossing once, until well browned and cooked
through. Transfer the baking pan to a wire rack and drizzle the vinegar
over the hot ingredients. Stir well to scrape up any browned bits in the
pan. Cool for a couple of minutes before serving.

Pork and Pineapple Kebabs with Fresh Salsa

Makes 4 servings

Ingredients:

1 pound pork tenderloin, halved lengthwise and each piece cut into
    8 equal sections (for a total of 16 pieces)
2 teaspoons purchased jerk seasoning blend
Twelve 1½-inch chunks of peeled and cored pineapple
Nonstick cooking spray
1 large red or orange bell pepper, stemmed, cored, and finely chopped
¼ cup minced red onion
12 grape tomatoes, chopped
2 tablespoons purchased pickled jalapeño rings, chopped
1½ tablespoons fresh lime juice

Directions:

Put the pork pieces in a large bowl, add the jerk seasoning blend, and
toss until the meat is well and evenly coated.

Thread the pork and pineapple pieces onto four 10-inch bamboo
skewers, starting and ending with a piece of pork on each skewer,
using 4 pieces of pork and 3 pieces of pineapple on each skewer.

Coat a grill pan with nonstick cooking spray and warm it over
medium-high heat. Add the skewers and cook for 12 to 15 minutes,
turning once, or until an instant-read meat thermometer inserted into
a piece of pork registers 145°F for a pink, hot center or 155°F for well-
done pork.

To make the salsa, mix the bell pepper, onion, tomatoes, jalapeño,
and lime juice in a small serving bowl.

Transfer the skewers to a serving platter. Serve the salsa along
with the skewers.

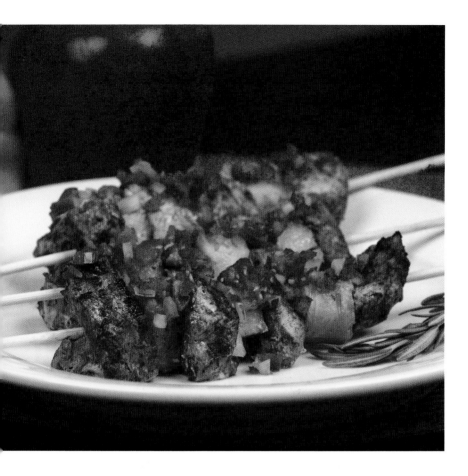

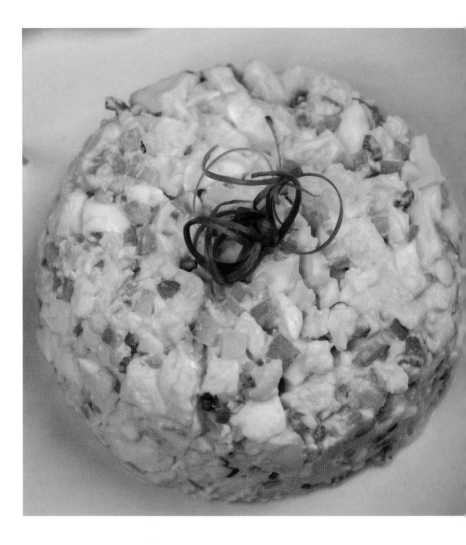

Enlightened Egg Salad

Makes 3 servings

Ingredients:

6 large eggs
1/3 cup soft silken tofu
1 1/2 tablespoons apple cider vinegar
1 teaspoon prepared yellow mustard
1 teaspoon jarred white horseradish
1/2 teaspoon table salt
2 medium celery ribs, finely diced
2 medium scallions, trimmed and thinly sliced

Directions:

Set the eggs in a large saucepan, fill it two-thirds full of water, and bring it to a boil over high heat. Boil for 4 minutes, then remove the saucepan from the heat. Cover and set aside for 5 minutes.

Gently drain the eggs into a colander set in the sink. Rinse with cold water until room temperature, then peel the eggs.

Split 3 eggs in half through the more pointed ends and remove the yolks. Discard these yolks or save them for another use.

Put these egg whites and the remaining whole eggs in a medium bowl. Use a fork to lightly mash the eggs, leaving larger pieces intact for texture.

Put the tofu, vinegar, mustard, horseradish, and salt in a mini food processor or a small blender; cover and process until smooth. Alternatively, press these ingredients through a fine-mesh strainer, then stir the mixture well to create a creamy sauce.

Pour this sauce over the eggs. Add the celery and scallions. Stir gently but well until evenly combined. Serve at once or cover and store in the fridge for up to 2 days.

Oven-Fried Cod Cakes

Makes 2 servings

Ingredients:

One 10-ounce cod fillet

½ cup shredded packed zucchini, squeezed dry by the handful

½ cup loosely packed, peeled, and shredded sweet potato

6 tablespoons almond flour

½ teaspoon dried thyme

½ teaspoon onion powder

½ teaspoon table salt

½ teaspoon ground black pepper

Several dashes hot red pepper sauce, such as sriracha or Tabasco sauce

Nonstick cooking spray

Directions:

Position the rack in the oven's center and heat the oven to 400°F. Line a lipped baking sheet with parchment paper or a silicone baking mat.

Bring a large saucepan of water to a simmer over high heat. Slip the fillet into the water, reduce the heat, and poach for 5 minutes. Gently drain the cod into a colander set in the sink or use a slotted spoon to transfer the fillet to a medium bowl. Cool for 5 minutes, then flake the cod with a fork.

Stir in the zucchini, sweet potato, almond flour, thyme, onion powder, salt, pepper, and hot pepper sauce until uniform. Use cleaned hands to form this mixture into four 4-inch patties, a scant ½ cup per patty (which will then be a little thick, like hockey pucks).

Set the patties on the prepared baking sheet and spray them with nonstick cooking spray. Bake for 15 to 20 minutes, until lightly browned and crisp at the edges. Cool for a couple of minutes before serving hot.

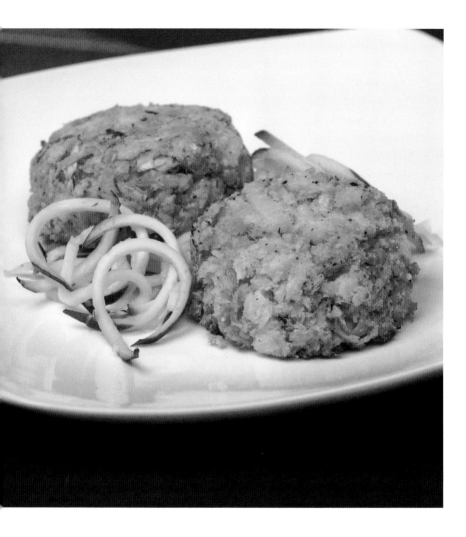

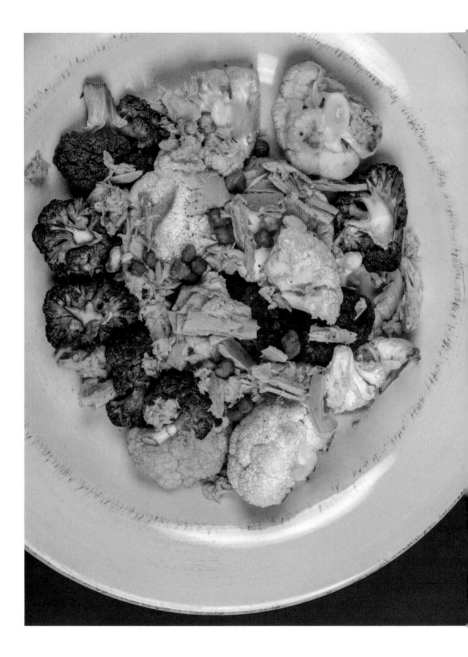

Warm Tuna with Roasted Cauliflower and Olives

Makes 2 servings

Ingredients:

4 cups cauliflower florets, chopped to bite size

1/4 cup sliced pitted green olives

Olive oil cooking spray

One 5-ounce can tuna packed in water, drained

2 tablespoons apple cider vinegar

1/2 teaspoon dried oregano

1/2 teaspoon red pepper flakes

1/4 teaspoon table salt

Directions:

Position the rack in the oven's center and heat the oven to 375°F.

Toss the cauliflower and olives in a small roasting pan or a lipped baking sheet. Lightly coat with olive oil spray.

Bake for 25 minutes, tossing twice, until the cauliflower is lightly browned, with crisp edges.

Remove the roasting pan or baking sheet from the oven. Flake the tuna over the cauliflower mixture; stir gently to combine. Set aside for 2 minutes to warm the tuna.

Sprinkle the vinegar, oregano, red pepper flakes, and salt over the tuna mixture. Toss gently but well to combine. Serve warm.

Apple-Almond Meatballs in an Herbed Tomato Sauce

Makes 4 servings

Ingredients:

1 pint (2 cups) grape tomatoes, halved

2 teaspoons minced peeled garlic

1 teaspoon table salt

1/2 teaspoon ground black pepper

Nonstick cooking spray

1 pound 93 percent lean ground beef

1/2 cup shredded fresh apple (about 1/2 a medium apple)

2 tablespoons almond flour

1 teaspoon smoked paprika

1 teaspoon dried oregano

1 teaspoon onion powder

Directions:

Position the rack in the oven's center and heat the oven to 375°F.

Place the tomatoes in a 9-x-13-inch baking pan. Add the minced garlic and 1/2 teaspoon salt and pepper; toss well. Spray the tomatoes with the nonstick cooking spray. Bake for 10 minutes.

Meanwhile, mix the ground beef, apple, almond flour, smoked paprika, oregano, onion powder, and 1/2 teaspoon salt in a medium bowl until evenly combined. Use cleaned hands to form this mixture into 12 meatballs, each made with a hefty 2 tablespoons.

When the tomatoes have baked for 10 minutes, set the meatballs among them and continue baking for 20 minutes, or until the meatballs have browned, the sauce is bubbling, and an instant-read meat thermometer inserted into the center of a meatball registers 165°F. Cool for a couple of minutes before serving warm.

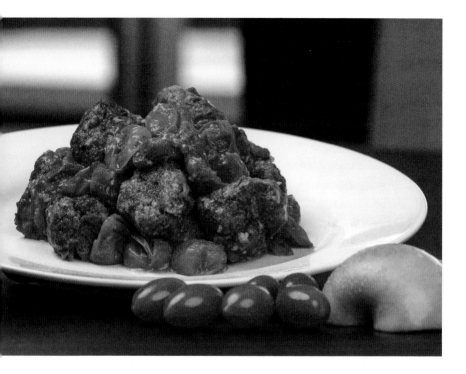

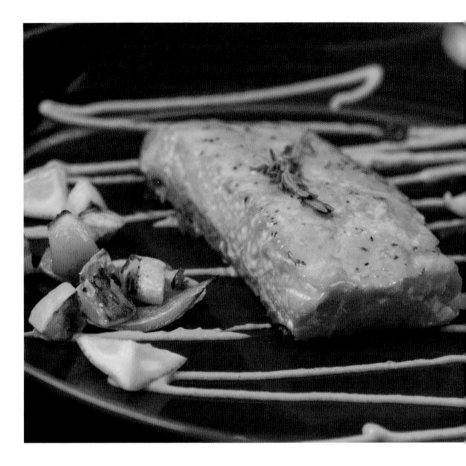

Sheet-Pan Salmon

Makes 2 servings

Ingredients:

24 ounces summer squash, cut into 1½-inch cubes (about 2 medium squash)

2 small red onions, trimmed, quartered, and broken up into pieces

½ teaspoon table salt

Nonstick cooking spray

Two 5-ounce skin-on salmon fillets

3 tablespoons Dijon mustard

½ teaspoon ground black pepper

Lemon wedges for garnishing

Directions:

Position the rack in the oven's center and heat the oven to 350°F.

Spread the squash and onions on a small, lipped sheet pan. Sprinkle with salt and coat with nonstick cooking spray. Toss well to coat. Bake for 15 minutes.

Increase the oven's temperature to 400°F. Smear the fillets with the mustard and sprinkle them with the pepper. Toss the vegetables in the pan, move them toward the edges to make room, and set the fillets skin-side down on the baking sheet.

Continue baking for 12 minutes, or until the salmon is cooked through. Squeeze a lemon wedge or two over everything and serve hot.

Warm Kale Salad with Chicken, Pine Nuts, and Tomatoes

Makes 2 servings

Ingredients:

4 cups loosely packed, chopped, stemmed curly-edged kale leaves

2 teaspoons olive oil

I tablespoon minced peeled garlic

I tablespoon pine nuts

6 ounces boneless skinless chicken breasts, cut into 1/2-inch pieces

1/2 teaspoon dried oregano

1/2 teaspoon mild smoked paprika

1/4 teaspoon table salt

2 small Roma or plum tomatoes, chopped (2/3 cup)

2 tablespoons white balsamic vinegar

Directions:

Place the kale in a large, heat-safe serving bowl.

Warm a medium nonstick skillet over medium heat. Add the oil, garlic, and pine nuts. Cook for I minute, stirring constantly, or until the pine nuts are lightly browned.

Add the chicken and cook for 3 to 4 minutes, stirring often, or until the chicken is cooked through and lightly browned.

Stir in the oregano, paprika, and salt until well combined. Stir in the tomatoes and cook for I minute, stirring often, or until warmed through.

Add the vinegar and cook until bubbling. Pour the contents of the salad over the kale and toss well.

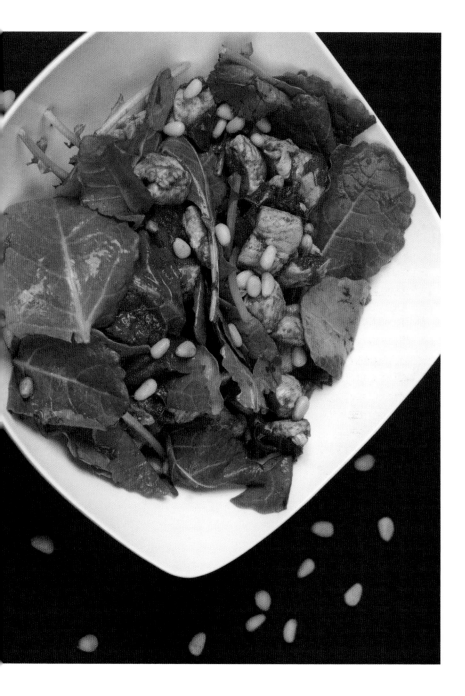

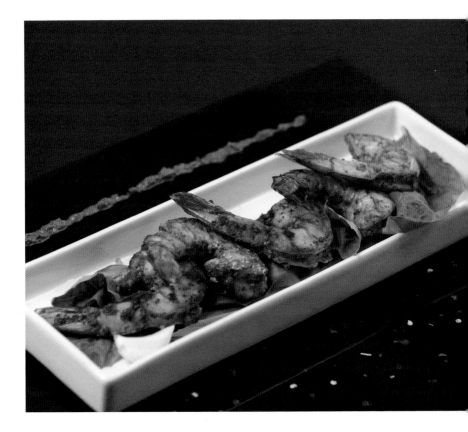

Herb Pesto Baked Shrimp

Makes 4 servings

Ingredients:

2 cups loosely packed fresh basil leaves

2 tablespoons chopped fresh chives or the green part of a scallion

2 tablespoons loosely packed fresh oregano leaves

I½ tablespoons olive oil

I tablespoon pine nuts

I tablespoon apple cider vinegar

I teaspoon minced peeled garlic

½ teaspoon red pepper flakes

½ teaspoon table salt

I¼ pounds (or 24) jumbo shrimp, peeled and deveined

Directions:

Position the rack in the oven's center and heat the oven to 375°F. Line a lipped baking sheet with parchment paper or a silicone baking mat.

Put the basil, chives or scallion, oregano, olive oil, pine nuts, vinegar, garlic, red pepper flakes, and salt in a food processor. Cover and process until smooth, stopping the machine at least once to scrape down the inside of the canister.

Scrape the basil mixture into a medium bowl. Add the shrimp and toss until well coated.

Place the shrimp about I inch apart on the prepared baking sheet. Divide any additional basil sauce among them. Bake for IO minutes, or until cooked through. Cool for 5 minutes before serving.

Spinach and Scallion Mini Muffins

Makes 2 servings (serving size is 3 muffins)

Ingredients:

Nonstick cooking spray

2 teaspoons olive oil

3 medium scallions, trimmed and thinly sliced

I cup packed baby spinach leaves, chopped

I large egg

2 tablespoons coconut flour

2 tablespoons almond flour

½ teaspoon baking powder

½ teaspoon table salt

¼ teaspoon ground black pepper

Directions:

Position the rack in the oven's center and heat the oven to 375°F. Lightly coat six indentations in a mini muffin pan with nonstick cooking spray.

Heat the oil in a small skillet set over medium heat. Add the scallions and spinach. Cook, stirring often, until the spinach wilts and the mixture is aromatic, about 2 minutes. Remove the skillet from the heat; set aside for 5 minutes.

Scrape the contents of the skillet into a medium bowl. Stir in the egg until smooth, then stir in the coconut flour, almond flour, baking powder, salt, and pepper until uniform. Divide this mixture evenly among the prepared muffin tin indentations, about 2 tablespoons per indentation.

Bake for 20 minutes, or until puffed, set, and lightly browned. Cool on a wire rack in the tin for 5 minutes before unmolding and serving warm.

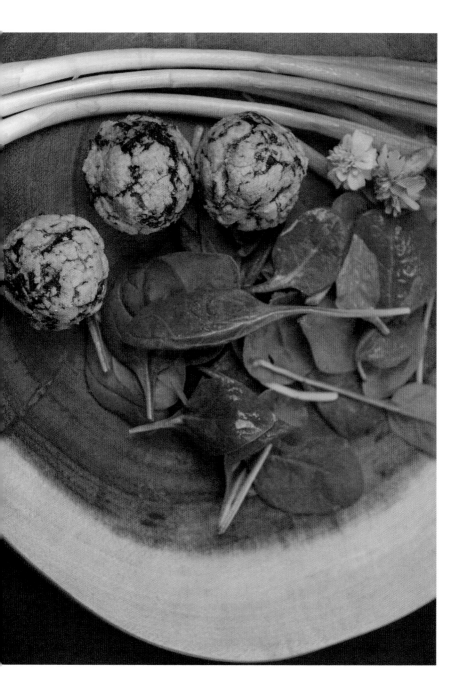

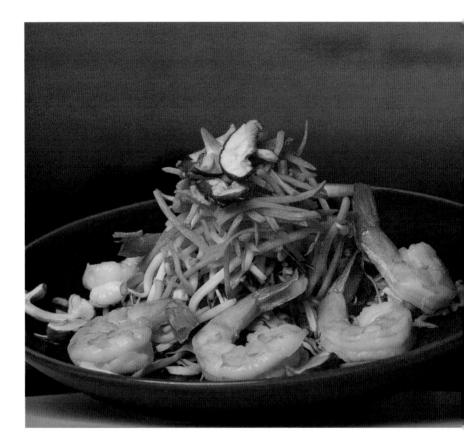

Shrimp Egg Roll Salad

Makes 1 serving

Ingredients:

2 tablespoons apple cider vinegar

2 teaspoons low-sodium soy sauce

1 teaspoon ketchup

1 teaspoon natural-style creamy peanut butter

1 teaspoon bottled ginger juice

1 cup shredded, cored green cabbage

¼ cup bean sprouts

¼ cup shredded carrots

¼ cup sliced shiitake mushroom caps

5 ounces cooked cocktail shrimp

Sesame seeds for garnishing (optional)

Sriracha sauce for garnishing (optional)

Directions:

Whisk the vinegar, soy sauce, ketchup, peanut butter, and ginger juice in a small bowl until smooth.

Put the cabbage in a medium bowl and add 1 tablespoon of the vinegar dressing. Toss well to coat.

Mound the dressed cabbage in the center of a serving plate. Top with the bean sprouts, carrots, shiitakes, and shrimp. Make it pretty!

Drizzle the remaining dressing over the salad. If desired, sprinkle the sesame seeds over the salad and/or give it a squeeze of sriracha.

Super Simple Parmesan Pizza Chips

Makes 2 servings

Ingredients:

6 tablespoons finely shredded aged Parmigiano-Reggiano, found
in deli section (use finely shredded parmesan cheese as an
alternative)

½ teaspoon dried oregano

½ teaspoon ground black pepper

6 thin slices turkey pepperoni

Directions:

Position the rack in the oven's center and heat the oven to 350°F.
Line a small, lipped baking sheet with parchment paper or a silicone
baking mat.

Use 1 tablespoon of grated cheese each to make 6 small mounds on
the prepared baking sheet. Sprinkle the mounds with the oregano and
pepper. Set a slice of pepperoni on top of each.

Bake for 8 minutes, or until melted and lightly browned. Cool for
5 minutes. (They must cool to crisp and set.) Gently blot off any
excess grease with a paper towel. Serve warm or at room temperature.

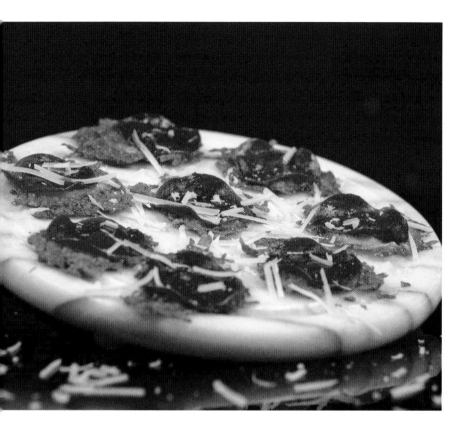

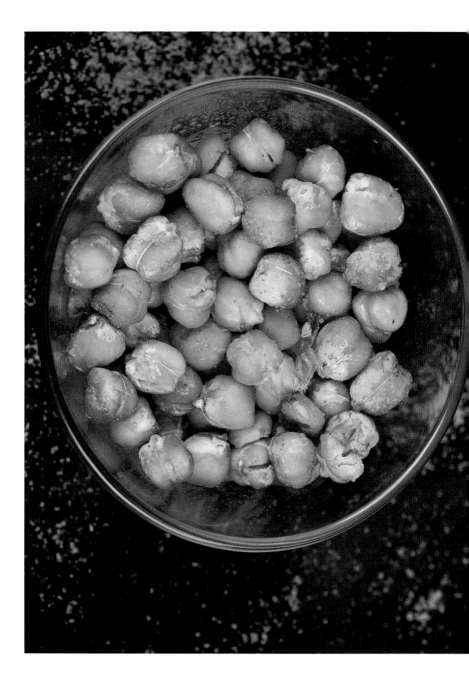

Crispy Curried Chickpeas

Makes 4 servings

Ingredients:

One 15-ounce can chickpeas, drained, rinsed, and patted dry

2 teaspoons olive oil

1½ teaspoons yellow curry powder

1 teaspoon white wine vinegar

¼ teaspoon table salt

Directions:

Position the rack in the oven's center and heat the oven to 375°F. Line a small, lipped baking sheet with parchment paper or a silicone baking mat.

Mix the chickpeas, oil, curry powder, vinegar, and salt in a medium bowl until the chickpeas are thoroughly and evenly coated. Spread them in one layer on the prepared baking sheet.

Bake for 45 minutes, or until crispy. Transfer the baking sheet to a wire rack and cool for 5 minutes. Serve warm.

Spicy Asparagus Spears with Turkey Bacon

Makes 4 servings

Ingredients:

8 slices turkey bacon, preferably uncured

1½ teaspoons salt-free chili powder

8 thin asparagus spears, trimmed of tough, woody ends

Nonstick cooking spray

Directions:

Position the rack in the oven's center and heat the oven to 375°F.

Sprinkle the slices of bacon with the chili powder. One at a time, roll a slice of bacon around an asparagus spear, starting at the bottom and winding the bacon up until the spear is covered.

Coat a small, lipped baking sheet with nonstick cooking spray. Lay the spears on the sheet with ½ inch between each. Lightly coat the bacon-wrapped spears with nonstick cooking spray.

Bake for 20 minutes, or until the bacon is crisp and cooked through. Transfer the baking sheet to a wire rack and cool for at least 5 minutes before serving. Serve warm or at room temperature.

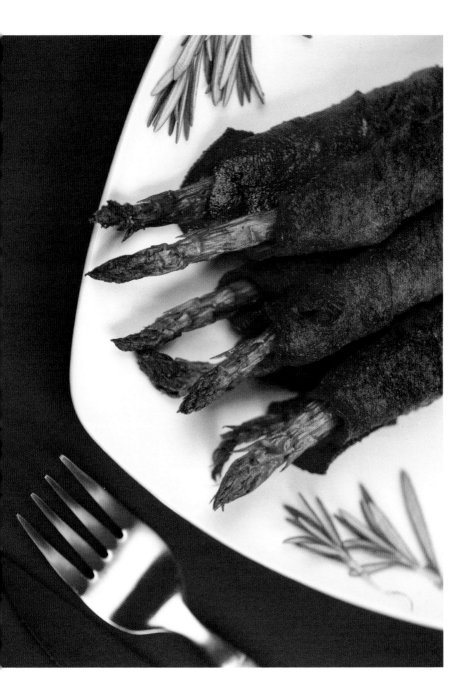

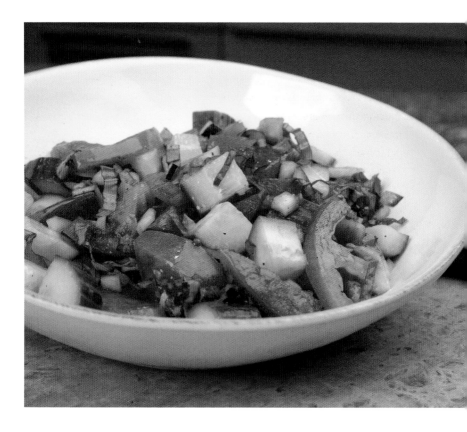

Cucumber Tomato Salad

Makes 2 servings

Ingredients:

5 cups whole tomatoes (any of your choice)

2 medium cucumbers

I tablespoon red wine vinegar

2 tablespoons extra-virgin olive oil

¼ red onion, finely chopped

¼ teaspoon fresh basil, chopped

Salt and pepper

Directions:

Chop the tomatoes and cucumbers into small, bite-size pieces and combine in a bowl.

In a separate bowl, combine the vinegar, olive oil, onion, and basil.

Add salt and pepper to taste.

Pour the oil mixture over the tomatoes and serve.

White Bean Hummus

Makes 2 servings

Ingredients:

One 15-ounce can cannellini beans, drained and rinsed

3 tablespoons unfiltered apple cider vinegar

2 tablespoons tahini

1 medium garlic clove, peeled

½ teaspoon table salt

1 tablespoon minced, stemmed, seeded canned chipotle chili in adobo
   sauce

Directions:

Put all the ingredients in a food processor. Cover and process until smooth, stopping the machine once to scrape down the inside of the canister. If the hummus is too thick, add water in 1-tablespoon increments to get the consistency you like.

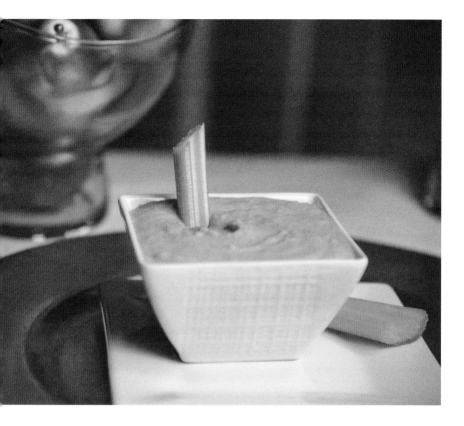

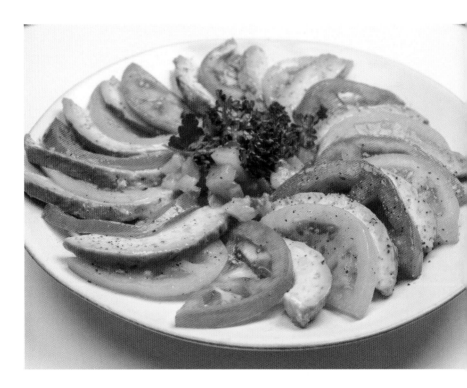

Tomato Avocado Salad

Makes 2 servings

Ingredients:

I red tomato

I yellow tomato

I avocado

Preferred seasoning of your choice

Directions:

Cut tomatoes and avocados into thin slices and spread out on a plate.

Add your preferred seasoning to taste.

Air-Fried Avocado

Makes 2 servings

For those with an air fryer, these are a delicious treat!

Ingredients:

1 firm avocado, peeled, cut in half, pit removed

Salt and pepper

Garlic salt (optional)

Seasoned gluten-free bread crumbs or whole-wheat bread crumbs

Olive oil spray (optional)

Directions:

Season the avocado with salt and pepper; garlic salt is okay too.

Press the avocado halves into the seasoned bread crumbs on all sides so that the avocado is fully coated.

You can mist with an olive oil spray, but it's optional.

Place the avocado halves in the air fryer basket and cook them at 375°F for 7 to 8 minutes. Then move the hot avocados to a plate and enjoy!

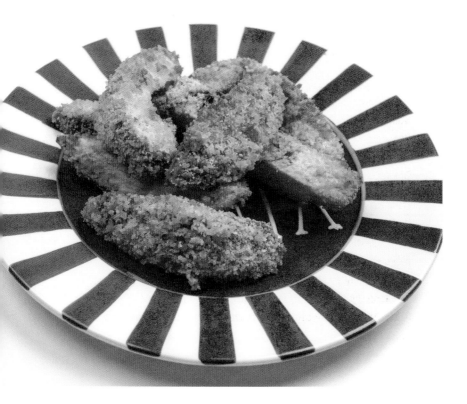

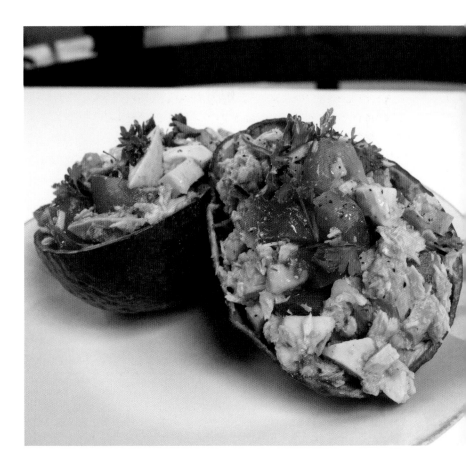

Tuna Avocado Boats

Makes 2 servings

Ingredients:

I avocado, cut in half, pit removed, diced, skins reserved

One 5-ounce can low-sodium tuna packed in water, drained

½ tomato, diced (about 3 tablespoons)

I stalk celery, chopped (about 3 tablespoons)

Small handful parsley, chopped (about 2 tablespoons)

Juice from ½ a lemon

Directions:

In a small bowl, combine all the ingredients and mix them together with a fork. Really smash the avocado to break it up.

Divide the mixture between the 2 avocado skins and serve.

Deviled Avocado Eggs

Makes 3 servings

Ingredients:

6 large hard-boiled eggs

2 teaspoons white vinegar

¼ cup pureed avocado

Dash salt and black pepper

Dash nutmeg (optional)

Directions:

Peel the shell off the hard-boiled eggs and rinse. Cut the eggs in half lengthwise.

Remove the egg yolks and place them in a small bowl.

On a platter, place the egg whites in a circle and set to the side.

Add vinegar, pureed avocado, salt, and black pepper to the egg yolks.

Using a fork, mix all the ingredients together until the egg yolks are smooth and creamy; spoon into each of the egg whites.

Sprinkle the eggs with nutmeg (optional) and serve immediately.

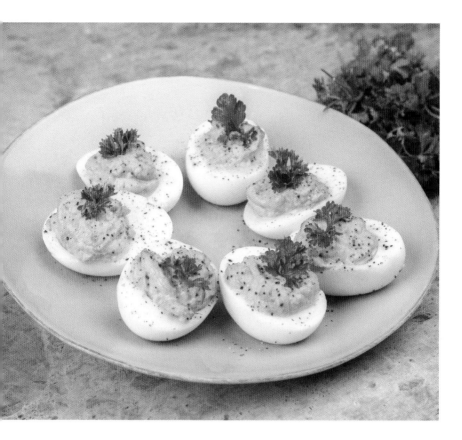

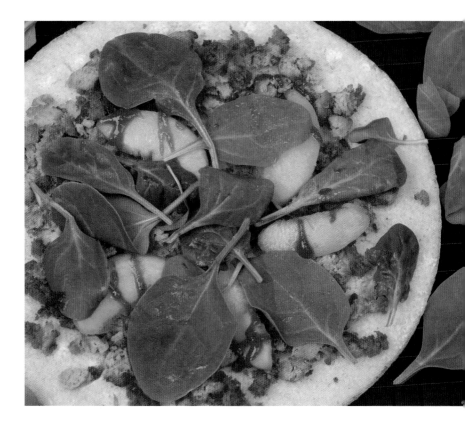

Cauliflower Flatbread

Makes 2 servings (Serving size: half a flatbread)

Ingredients:

One 10-inch plain cauliflower pizza crust

8 ounces Italian-style chicken or turkey sausage, any casings
    removed

1 large ripe peach, halved, pitted, thinly sliced

1 cup baby spinach leaves, packed

1 tablespoon balsamic vinegar (or white balsamic vinegar for a sweeter
    flavor)

Up to 2 teaspoons sriracha sauce

Directions:

Position the rack in the oven's center and heat the oven to 375°F. Set
the pizza crust on a large baking sheet (preferably a lipped sheet).

Warm a medium nonstick skillet over medium heat. Crumble in the
chicken sausage and cook, stirring often, for 3 minutes or until lightly
browned.

Spread the cooked sausage around the crust, leaving a ½-inch
border all around the edge. Top with the peach slices. Bake for
15 minutes, or until the crust is crisp.

Meanwhile, toss the spinach and balsamic vinegar in a medium
bowl until well coated.

When the pizza is ready, transfer the baking sheet to a wire rack.
While the pizza is hot, drizzle the sriracha over it, then top with the
dressed spinach. Cool for a minute or two before slicing into wedges
and serving.

CHAPTER 7

JJ's Personal Tips for Success

Here are a few tips that will help you be successful!

Find your tribe and join our Facebook group.

I want to emphasize how important it is to join our Facebook community of 850,000 people. This is your tribe of like-minded folks trying to lose weight and get healthy. When trying to make a lifestyle change, you must lean on a tribe for support. Don't try to do this alone. Struggles and challenges will arise, but the support group helps you persevere. The social connection keeps you accountable and inspires you to continue forward. Together we all win.

It's so easy to trick yourself into thinking you can do it all alone. And, quite frankly, in the beginning, you probably can. But when you fall off the wagon or feel weak or frustrated, support groups help you push through and continue forward. I have coached tens of thousands of folks trying to lose weight and get healthy, and they all needed support at some point along their journey. So, rely on the Facebook support group, as this is your tribe. They are there to help you. I am there to help you. Get support, encouragement, and tips from me and others at https://www.facebook.com/groups/Green.Smoothie .Cleanse/.

Prepare to be uncomfortable.

For the first few days, you will feel hungry and irritable. Don't worry about that, and don't be afraid of those feelings. You have to focus on getting your body through this process if you stand any chance of breaking unhealthy eating habits. Your body has the natural ability to maintain your ideal weight if you focus on getting healthy. As the days go on, you will want less food and will learn to eat in moderation. You are training your body to have better eating habits. So go through the process, be uncomfortable from time to time, and let your body reward you for it in the end. Many of us eat out of habit and boredom—that's called emotional hunger, not physical hunger. This is a perfect time to learn the difference between the two.

Expect your weight to fluctuate.

While detoxing, you may gain on some days, while other days you may lose weight. This is perfectly normal. Weight fluctuates due to three things in the body: muscle, fat, and water. Muscle weighs the most—that's why you can work out and build muscle and thereby *gain* weight. But you're actually making progress by building muscle because it will help you burn fat all day long.

For women, water is the biggest culprit, due to our hormones. Many of us gain five to ten pounds of water weight during our cycle. For some, excess salt/sodium causes water to be trapped under the tissues in the body, making us weigh more and look bloated and puffy! So, don't sweat it if your weight loss is a little up and down. Make sure you're paying attention to your measurements, your before photos, and how you're actually feeling! When it's up every week, week after week, then you know you have a problem! Also, look into getting a Tanita scale—it will tell you your weight and the percentage of muscle, fat, and water in your body. This is helpful for people who work out!

Drink more water than you usually do.

Throughout this program you should plan on drinking a lot more water than you typically do. This is due to the fact that carbs tend to cause your body to hold on to water, and when you reduce the amount of carbs, your body will begin to release the extra water. So, you will need to replace this water. You may even experience dry mouth when you begin this program. A general guide is to try to get at least half your body weight in ounces of water daily. For example, if you weigh 160 pounds, you should drink at least eighty ounces of water per day. If you follow a detox program, you may need up to a gallon per day. One habit to maintain is to drink a glass of water when you wake up to hydrate your body from overnight and to set the tone for more water to come throughout the day. You can also slowly drink a glass of water or some coffee once you start feeling hungry. Often by the time you've finished your drink, your hunger will have passed.

Preparation is key to success.

It's important to spend some time preparing for success. This includes reading this book, completing grocery shopping for food and supplements, and gaining the support you need from family and friends. These activities will make the cleanse easier and ensure you get the best results.

Make your health a priority.

You must begin thinking differently. First, decide that your health is one of the top priorities in your life. You deserve to live a healthy life. If you prepare your mind and absorb the knowledge offered to you in this book, you will have all the power you need to become your best self and transform your life in every way. Even if you are a busy mom or high-powered career executive, know that today begins the journey toward your most amazing, beautiful self. It is time to treat your body as the greatest gift that you have. It is time to shine as the person you were always meant to be. When you have healthy and positive energy in life, amazing things like love, joy, success, and wealth come your way. Every interaction at work, church, home, or in the streets can be simply magnetic. Get healthy, lose weight, and watch your entire life begin to change for the better.

Get support from family and friends.

Our eating habits are greatly influenced by our culture and by family and friends. Think about the people you eat with most often: loved ones, friends, and lovers. For a lot of us, food equals fun. We eat to socialize, celebrate, and show love to one another. How many people eat right until they get around their family and friends? Our family and friends have the strongest

JJ'S PERSONAL TIPS FOR SUCCESS **143**

influence on how successful we will be in changing our habits and living a healthy lifestyle. They often encourage us to indulge or tell us we look good and don't need to be on a diet.

Whenever we tell someone we love that we are making some changes and getting healthier, their response will have a great effect on whether we succeed or fail. Studies show that people who don't get support from loved ones are less successful in achieving their life goals. When you communicate to a family member that you're trying to lose weight, it is essential that they show support and encouragement and that they understand that your new lifestyle is important to you. If they do the opposite or criticize your food choices, you will have a harder time succeeding, and this disagreement will become a source of stress and tension in the relationship. The most ideal situation is when a family member decides to change their behavior along with you. That way, you can hold each other accountable. If that's not your experience, it's even more important that you find a community that will support you in this journey.

Detox family and friends.

Sometimes you need to detox your emotions as well as your body by withdrawing from family and friends who discourage you or tell you "You can't do it" or "You're not ready to do it," blah blah blah! If there is negative talk coming from some people in your life, I would encourage you to limit the amount of time you spend with them. We all have enough negative thoughts on our own without people adding to them! Don't gravitate to people who tell you you can't do something. Know that when you start this cleanse, you will want to give up. It's normal. But I know that sometimes the only way to grow in life is to be uncomfortable. How else do you grow mentally, spiritually, and physically? When you cheat or mess up, it's no big deal. I guarantee you that if you cheat a little bit one day on the cleanse, you are still eating better than you've been eating most days prior to the cleanse. I call that progress! You are right where you're supposed to be on this journey! Uncomfortable, irritable, doubtful, cranky. And then one day, the joy, the energy, and the feeling of accomplishment settle in. Don't you want that feeling?

Take the time to address emotional eating.
During the 14-Day New Keto Cleanse, the restrictive regimen will be challenging if you struggle with emotional eating. This is a great time to address emotional eating and improve your relationship with food. It's important to process the uncomfortable emotions that drive many of us to try to self-soothe with food or other substances. This cleanse is a great opportunity to examine the roles that food plays in your life—not just for nourishment but to soothe or lessen your uncomfortable feelings. Not only can this cleanse help you break the habit of reaching for food to soothe, comfort, calm, or distract from unpleasant feelings but it's also a good time to think about new ways you can permanently process the roots of your emotional eating.

Sad or painful experiences are meant to teach us lessons we need to learn so that we can grow and mature—they are not meant to linger for years and years. Just as we can get rid of toxic waste from the body, we can get rid of toxic emotions. Instead of eating to distract ourselves from bad feelings, we need to process and eliminate them—just like the body does with food: it takes the nutrients it needs and expels the rest.

For more information on dealing with emotional eating, read my book *Think Yourself Thin: A 30-Day Guide to Permanent Weight Loss*. This book is dedicated to processing the feelings and struggles that have been keeping you from reaching your goal weight.

Engage in positive self-talk.

Thoughts and feelings turn into actions, and actions into reality. Remember, you are beginning a new chapter in your life. Let me encourage you right now to get started with your journey. Many ask, "How do I start?" or "How do I get there?" Well, it begins with positive self-talk. You want to stop thinking and saying negative things about yourself. You are not fat, lazy, ugly, or sick. Your true self is naturally thin, beautiful, and healthy. If you have negative thoughts about yourself, you'll attract negative people and outcomes in your life. If you say that you can never lose weight, you're exactly right: you won't. If you say you can, your subconscious mind believes that and begins to move your actions in the direction of losing weight.

Focus on getting healthy, and you'll never have to worry about weight again.

If you're just doing the cleanse for fast weight loss, you risk missing the additional benefits. Don't waste time being discouraged by the scale. Don't let the scale become your enemy! Focus on your overall health, and look at your energy level, sleep, and digestion for improvements. The long-term focus is on healthy living. Focus on getting healthy, and the weight loss will follow.

CHAPTER 8

How to Continue Losing Weight After the 14-Day New Keto Cleanse

Congratulations on taking control of your health by caring for your body and feeding it what it needs to be slim, healthy, and vibrant! You will reap the rewards now and continue to enjoy a lifestyle of optimal health and happiness. Be sure to always make time to nourish your inner spirit and soul by giving your body the rest and relaxation it needs to stay strong and healthy. You have given yourself a wonderful gift of optimal health and wellness.

Continuing to Lose Weight After the New Keto Cleanse

Normal weight loss of about one to two pounds per week is very healthy! This cleanse should give you a ten- to fifteen-pound jump-start on your weight loss to get you motivated to continue.

After the 14-Day New Keto Cleanse, you can do the following:

- Continue the 14-Day New Keto Cleanse for life. You can continue the plan as designed and just alternate the keto smoothie recipes and low-carb, fat-burning recipes throughout the month. You can also continue intermittent fasting and Tabata. Feel free to increase your workout routine as you desire.

- Continue rotating the New Keto Cleanse, Green Smoothie Cleanse, and Apple Cider Vinegar Cleanse throughout the month.
- Adopt the DHEMM System, my permanent weight-loss system, detailed in the *Green Smoothies for Life* book.
- Join my VIP program, Slay at Any Age, if you need additional support and accountability. You will experience learning, joy, inspiration, personal growth, and empowerment. Together, we'll take back control of our health and our lives! I share strategies, tips, healthy recipes, detox methods, and many other topics that help you stay committed to living your best life. Join at www.JJSmithOnline.com.

My Other Popular Detox Programs

10-Day Green Smoothie Program

The Green Smoothie Cleanse (GSC) is a ten-day detox/cleanse made up of green leafy veggies, fruit, and water. Green smoothies are filling and healthy, and you will enjoy drinking them. Your body will also thank you for drinking them.

The 10-Day Green Smoothie Program can be done as either the full or modified cleanse. You can learn about the Green Smoothie Cleanse in the books *10-Day Green Smoothie Cleanse* and *Green Smoothies for Life*. There are over one hundred green smoothie recipes in the books.

You can expect to lose some weight, increase your energy levels, reduce your cravings, clear your mind, and improve your digestion and overall health. It is an experience that could change your life if you stick with it.

7-Day Apple Cider Vinegar Cleanse

The 7-Day Apple Cider Vinegar (ACV) Cleanse is another revolutionary cleanse that includes meals and drinks that help support the body's natural detoxification process and promote a healthy environment for good bacteria in the body.

The 7-Day ACV Cleanse involves consuming apple cider vinegar for six days, along with "fasting with food" and using the seventh day as a transition day to break the cleanse. Instead of abstaining from food completely like in a traditional fast or water fast, you eat small amounts of food in a way that produces the therapeutic benefits of fasting—increased fat burning, lower blood-sugar levels, and reduced inflammation—but without the hunger. The healthy menu is low in carbs and protein but higher in fat. Your body stays nourished while also gaining the benefits of fasting. Long-term fasting can be harmful, but this seven-day cleanse is safe and effective.

The DHEMM System

My DHEMM System is a lifestyle for permanent weight loss. The DHEMM System is a breakthrough permanent weight loss solution that helps you detoxify, cleanse, and burn body fat naturally. You can learn the entire DHEMM System in my *Green Smoothies for Life* book.

The DHEMM System stands for the following:

- **Detox:** Use one of the many detox methods available. I teach twenty-one detox methods in the VIP program.

- **Hormonal Balance:** Optimize your hormones for weight loss.
- **Eat Clean:** Eat healthy, whole, and unprocessed foods.
- **Mental Mastery:** Achieve the right mental focus to stay motivated. Gain mental mastery.
- **Move:** Get moving and increase your physical activity.

If Weight Loss Stalls

If you begin to plateau and weight loss stalls (if two weeks have gone by and you haven't lost any more weight), I know exactly what you have to do next: Check your hormones. If you have stubborn body fat that isn't responding to healthy eating, then hormones are the likely culprit. In my bestseller *Lose Weight Without Dieting or Working Out!*, I have two chapters titled "Correct Hormonal Imbalances" and "Stop Weight Gain During Perimenopause and Menopause" that explain the six hormones that cause weight gain by slowing your metabolism and preventing your body from losing weight.

It is essential to understand the role hormones play in how we gain and lose weight. Some hormones tell you you're hungry, some tell you you're full; some tell your body what to do with the food that is eaten, whether to use it as fuel for energy or store it as fat, which causes us to gain weight. Hormones are responsible for metabolizing fat. By controlling your hormones, you can control your weight.

Hormones affect how you feel, how you look, and, most important, how you maintain your weight and health. When your hormones are balanced properly, you will have great health, beauty, and vibrancy. When your hormones are imbalanced, you have mood swings, you crave unhealthy foods, and you feel sluggish and lethargic. Hormones are critical to weight loss, and balancing them will help you stay slim and healthy.

Best and Worst Keto Foods to Eat

If your goal is to maintain a healthy, keto-friendly diet that goes beyond the recipes in this book, there are some key foods to consider avoiding, and others to think about integrating more into your diet. As a general guideline for grocery shopping, here are the best keto-friendly foods to stock up on to help you stay in fat-burning mode. This is not a complete, exhaustive list but a general one that you can use as a guide.

Foods to Eat

Carbs

- Asparagus
- Bell peppers
- Berries (blueberry, raspberry, blackberry)
- Broccoli
- Brussels sprouts
- Cauliflower
- Celery
- Cucumber
- Eggplant
- Green beans
- Kale
- Lemons and limes
- Spinach

- Tomatoes
- Zucchini

Protein
- Beef
- Chicken
- Eggs
- Fish, all types
- Lamb
- Natural cheeses
- Pork
- Salmon
- Sardines
- Sausages
- Seafood (lobster, shrimp, crab, etc.)
- Turkey
- Unsweetened, plain whole-milk Greek yogurt
- Venison
- Whole-milk ricotta or cottage cheese

Fats
- Avocado oil
- Avocados
- Butter
- Chia seeds
- Coconuts
- Flaxseeds
- Hemp hearts
- Nut butters, no sugar added
- Nuts

- Olive oil
- Olives
- Pumpkin seeds
- Sesame seeds

Foods to Avoid

Stay clear of these foods if you want to maintain a healthy keto lifestyle:

- Beans, peas, lentils, and peanuts
- Grains, such as rice, pasta, and oatmeal
- Low-fat dairy products
- Most alcohol, except whiskey, gin, tequila, rum, and vodka, which, when you drink them neat (straight with no mixers or chasers), are free of carbs
- Most fruits, except for lemons, limes, tomatoes, and berries
- Starchy vegetables, including corn and potatoes
- Refined white sugar
- Sugary beverages, including fruit juices and soda
- Trans fats, such as margarine or other hydrogenated fats
- Typical snack foods, such as potato chips, pretzels, and crackers

CHAPTER 9

Frequently Asked Questions (FAQs)

There are five categories of frequently asked questions. They are grouped as follows:

- how to succeed on the New Keto Cleanse program;
- what to eat or drink on the New Keto Cleanse program;
- getting in and out of ketosis;
- staying motivated and other tips;
- health, safety, and precautions.

How to Succeed on the New Keto Cleanse Program

How many carbs, fats, and proteins do I eat per day?
How many net carbs can I have per day?

This healthier version of keto (more flexible than the strict keto diet) consists of

- 10 percent carbs,
- 20 percent proteins, and
- 70 percent fats.

For weight loss, many recommend that you stay under twenty grams of net carbs per day on the standard keto diet.

However, this extremely low amount of carbs ultimately results in a rebound in weight gain and is not sustainable in the long run. Additionally, many people have too many cravings and give in to temptation when trying to be too strict and stay under twenty grams of net carbs. So it's possible to enjoy twenty to thirty grams of net carbs per day and still achieve your weight-loss goals. You could measure your blood ketones for a period of time to verify that up to thirty grams of net carbs per day still allows you to be successful on the program.

Do I need to count calories?

Because the focus of this program is not to restrict calorie intake, there is no need to count calories. As a general guideline, it will be important to focus on the amounts of macros (protein, fats, and carbs) you consume each day, with the most emphasis on staying under thirty grams of net carbs per day.

When do I need to eat?

You should eat within the eight-hour eating window on the 16:8 intermittent-fasting eating method. During that eight-hour window, enjoy the keto smoothies and low-carb, fat-burning meals and snacks. When you first begin, you will notice more hunger. Once your body adjusts to the program, your insulin levels will lower and your brain will stop signaling you to eat. In other words, the longer you stay on the program, the easier it becomes.

Can I have a "cheat day" on the New Keto Cleanse?
During the fourteen days, avoid cheat days and cheat meals altogether. They will slow your results. Every time you have a cheat day, you must begin the process of getting into ketosis all over again. After one cheat meal, it can take one to three days to get back into fat-burning mode. After the fourteen days, you can begin to add in cheat meals on occasion, and that won't undo most of your results.

Can I have healthy snacks on the New Keto Cleanse?
You should minimize snacking on the New Keto Cleanse. Having any food between your meals will raise your blood sugar levels, which raises your insulin levels. This will slow your ability to burn fat. It is a bad habit to eat all day. Rather, focus on eating for fuel. Then focus on other life priorities. You can enjoy one snack, which may include any veggies, peanut butter, almond butter, nuts and seeds, or any of the snack recipes included in this program. You should have no more than one snack during your eight-hour eating window. The goal is to eat snacks that are low in sugars and carbs.

Do I need to exercise on the New Keto Cleanse?
Exercise is fine on this program and is an important part of a healthy lifestyle. It's great for maintaining cardiovascular health and enhancing your moods. To begin with, I provide a simple, four-minute Tabata routine that will help accelerate your results. It's also important to listen to your body. If

you feel fatigued and need to rest when you first begin this program, that is perfectly fine also.

What to Eat or Drink on the New Keto Cleanse Program

What if I want to make my own healthy meals? Can I substitute any of the keto smoothies or meals in the plan?

If you want to make your own healthy meals, please ensure that they are clean, healthy, low-carb, and low-sugar meals. If you decide to customize week 1 or 2 of the meal plan, use the blank chart provided to write in the keto smoothies and meals you plan to eat. Remember, the shopping lists are for the designed plan. If you customize the plan, be sure to write a new shopping list that includes all the necessary ingredients.

Can you consume too much protein on keto?

This plan recommends a moderate amount of protein. As a general guideline, that is between three and six ounces of protein per meal, but the amounts can vary depending upon certain factors. As an example, if you work out or are younger, you will need more protein. So feel free to increase protein intake. Be sure you consume high-quality proteins such as lean red meats, fish, poultry, and eggs.

How will I consume that much fat each day?

Seventy percent of all of your calories should be from healthy fats. This might seem like a lot of fat, but what is important is that they are healthy fats that fuel the body. Examples of healthy fats include olive oil, MCT oil, wild-caught salmon, and nuts and seeds. You can also add healthy oils to most salads or foods as well.

Can I consume dairy, including cheese, on keto?

Yes, most dairy products are keto-friendly. Do choose full-fat dairy products such as butter, heavy cream, cheeses, and yogurts. The healthiest dairy products are organic, grass-fed dairy products. If you are allergic to dairy (including cheeses), then you should continue to avoid it, as usual.

Can I have regular coffee on the New Keto Cleanse? How much is too much?

Yes, you can enjoy coffee and tea on this program. However, drinking coffee throughout the day can increase your stress hormones, especially cortisol. This will interfere with sleep and make it more difficult to get into ketosis. Try to enjoy one cup of coffee per day or look to drink more decaf coffee and tea.

How can I avoid hidden carbs?

Hidden carbs are typically found in processed foods, drinks, sauces, and even many so-called sugar-free products. So, you must learn to read nutritional labels, focusing on calculating net carbs. To calculate net carbs, you take the total carbs and subtract fiber and sugar alcohols. Because fiber is a carbohydrate your body cannot digest, it passes through your digestive system unaltered. Also, sugar alcohols such as xylitol and erythritol are also indigestible, so they can be deducted from the total carb count as well. As an example, if the nutritional label says the following—total carbs fourteen grams, dietary fiber four grams, sugar alcohols six grams—then the net carbs would be four grams. Many products now provide the net carbs on the nutritional label as well.

Can I use salad dressing on the New Keto Cleanse?
Yes, you can have salad dressings if they have low-carb, low-sugar, keto-friendly ingredients. Be careful of store-bought salad dressings because they include a lot of hidden carbs that knock you out of ketosis. So be sure to read the label. Generally, any oil-based or vinaigrette dressing will be keto friendly.

Can I have diet drinks on the New Keto Cleanse?
The majority of diet drinks are fine on this program. Any diet drink with stevia, monk fruit, and sugar alcohols such as xylitol and erythritol are fine. Diet drinks with aspartame or saccharin aren't as healthy but generally won't knock you out of ketosis.

When can I enjoy breads again?
Traditional bread, including whole grain and whole-wheat bread, is too high in carbohydrates to include on the New Keto Cleanse. There are, however, many low-carb, keto-friendly alternatives on the market today that you could try.

Can I use agave or honey instead of stevia in the smoothies?

Agave is okay in moderation, but if you're interested in weight loss, stevia and monk fruit are the number-one sweeteners. The way to think about sweeteners is how much they cause insulin spikes, because that determines how much they will cause fat storage in the body. Foods are given glycemic index (GI) ratings according to how much they cause insulin spikes. Stevia and monk fruit are a 0 (which is ideal). Agave is a 20. Honey is about a 30. Brown sugar/raw sugar is a 65. And white refined sugar is an 80. So that gives you some perspective. I have four friends who all use different brands of stevia, and none of us like the others' stevia because they all taste different. If you think you don't like stevia, perhaps just try another brand.

Can I have alcohol on the New Keto Cleanse?

Limit your alcohol on this program. If you're able to, completely avoid it for the first two weeks. When alcohol is present in your system, it stops your cells from burning ketones as fuel. In other words, you won't be burning stored body fat. Alcohol slows your weight loss with virtually every weight-loss plan. For the long term, you can learn to enjoy keto-friendly drinks, such as neat tequila, rum and diet coke, and many others.

Getting Into and Out of Ketosis

How long does it take to get into ketosis?

It depends on the individual. Some folks can enter ketosis overnight, whereas others might take a month or longer to get into fat-burning mode. Scientists say the shift from using glucose to breaking down stored fat as a source of energy usually begins over two to four days of eating fewer than twenty to fifty grams of carbohydrates per day. However, everyone is different, and this time frame may be longer for some.

Should I test for ketosis with keto strips? What if my ketones no longer show up in my urine?

You can use keto urine strips to measure ketones. There are many people who do this in the beginning. Ideally, once your system is using up all the ketones, however, you will no longer have ketones in your urine. That doesn't mean you aren't in ketosis; it just means you're using up all your ketones for fuel—which means it's working.

You can measure your level of ketosis through over-the-counter urine tests (keto sticks), but don't get fixated on the results. Pay attention to whether you're losing fat and feeling more energy and better mental clarity, all positive signs you are in ketosis. I have seen folks get disappointed by the results on the keto stick when their scale clearly indicated they were losing weight. Don't fall into this trap. Focus on the results you're getting, not just the keto stick.

Will lemon water knock me out of ketosis?

You can have as much lemon water as you want as long as you don't add sugar. If you want to sweeten it, feel free to add stevia or monk fruit.

Will bone broth knock me out of ketosis?

Bone broth should be consumed during your eating window only. It is like consuming food or other broths or soups and will stop ketosis for a short period of time. So it's safer to drink only during your eating window.

Will monk fruit or stevia knock me out of ketosis?

No, monk fruit or stevia should not affect ketosis. There are relatively insignificant changes to your blood sugar levels when you consume monk fruit or stevia.

Will chewing gum knock me out of ketosis?

No, but always choose sugar-free gum.

Staying Motivated and Other Tips

How is this program different from the 10-Day Green Smoothie Cleanse (GSC)?

GSC is a very effective detox that will jump-start weight loss. However, the New Keto Cleanse is designed more specifically for burning fat, lowering your sugar consumption, and achieving sustainable weight loss. It features keto smoothies, which are low in carbs and sugar, fat-burning meals, and other lifestyle habits that put the body into fat-burning mode. So, the New Keto Cleanse is an effective weight-loss plan that will help you burn fat faster, all while enjoying savory meals.

If I just finished the 10-Day Green Smoothie Cleanse, can I still do the 14-Day New Keto Cleanse?

After either the 10-Day Green Smoothie Cleanse or the 7-Day Apple Cider Vinegar Cleanse, you can begin the New

Keto Cleanse right away; it is a plan that can be followed for life.

What if I don't want to lose weight?

This plan is still great for anyone looking to achieve the health benefits of New Keto Cleanse. This program promotes health and longevity by reducing inflammation and reversing many ailments and diseases we struggle with as we age. This program is about maintaining a healthy body for life.

How long will my smoothie keep?

To ensure you get maximum taste and nutrition, it is always ideal to drink your smoothie the same day you blend it. However, if you are busy or for some other reason can't make your smoothies fresh, then they can keep extremely well for up to two days in the refrigerator. A glass jar with a lid is ideal to safely store your smoothies. Covering your smoothies with a tight lid minimizes oxidation and absorption of other smells from the refrigerator. Additionally, making the smoothies the night before is okay if it helps you stay on track.

Health, Safety, and Precautions

Should I take my medications or supplements during the New Keto Cleanse?

You should never stop taking any medications prescribed by a doctor. I am not a medical doctor, so you should consult with your doctor prior to starting this program.

Can you do the New Keto Cleanse while pregnant or breastfeeding?

This is a nutrient-rich meal plan with adequate nutrition for most. In chapter 3, I have a section detailing who this program is not ideal for. You will want to make sure the healthier version of keto, combined with intermittent fasting, is safe for you and your child while pregnant or breastfeeding, so I suggest you consult with your doctor prior to starting this program.

Can children do the New Keto Cleanse?

This plan includes a lot of lean protein, good carbs, and healthy fats, so there's no reason a child could not benefit from the healthy diet it provides. Because intermittent fasting limits the eating window to eight hours, you will need to evaluate if two meals or two meals and a snack is adequate for your child. For that reason, I suggest you consult with your doctor prior to putting your child on this program.

Aren't saturated fats bad for me?

One of the common mistakes people make when following the keto lifestyle is eating too many saturated and trans fats. Although the keto diet is a high-fat diet, the majority of the fats should be healthy fats, which are monounsaturated fats and polyunsaturated fats. They raise your "good" cholesterol levels, so feel free to enjoy them. They include avocado, wild-caught salmon, olives, nuts and seeds, olive oil, MCT oil, and coconut butter. You will want to limit your intake of trans fat and saturated fat; it can increase your "bad" cholesterol and put you at risk of heart disease. Examples of trans fats and saturated fats to avoid include vegetable oils, fried foods, canola oil, and margarine.

Will my cholesterol go up on the New Keto Cleanse?

The real culprits behind high cholesterol levels are sugars and carbs. Your cholesterol levels should stabilize on this program. When you first begin this program, you can expect cholesterol levels to increase for a short time. After that, though, they should normalize and stay at healthy levels.

Can I do the New Keto Cleanse if I don't have a gallbladder?

If you don't have a gallbladder, you may experience incomplete digestion of all the fats and so could experience more bloating, nausea, and right-shoulder pain on this program. You would likely need some purified bile salts to help promote healthy bile levels so you don't experience any pain or symptoms. Be sure to consult with your doctor to get approval before starting this program if you don't have a gallbladder.

CHAPTER 10

Testimonials

Here are just a few of the testimonials from those who have done the 14-Day New Keto Cleanse.

I have lost 15 pounds! My energy is through the roof and the discipline is on point. I have fallen in love with intermittent fasting again. I have also enjoyed the keto recipes . . . and Tabata! Thank you so much for this cleanse!

—LaKesha M.

I have lost 10 pounds and inches all over and am so proud of myself. I love the keto recipes and can continue doing this forever. Thank you, JJ!!

—Bernadette R.

I have lost 11 pounds and some inches. My energy has increased. I remained very disciplined throughout the cleanse. I will continue with the intermittent fasting forever. And I am able to wear my wedding ring without forcing it for the first time in close to a year. I am proud of me!

—Alicia A.

I have lost 12 pounds and many inches. My energy level has skyrocketed and I'm so motivated to do meal preps. The fat-burning meals are amazing, the keto smoothies are so filling, and I find that I'm drinking more water as a result of intermittent fasting. This program is so easy to follow and stay on.

—*Sam R.*

I lost inches and 10 pounds. My energy is a lot better. I feel lighter. I could have done better with the Tabata workouts and drinking water, but I injured my shoulder and back. The eating was great and I LOVE the recipes—ready to jump back in and start over!

—*Maxy M.*

I lost 12 pounds and 2 inches off my waist and thighs. I had to go to the office on Friday. It's a 2½ block walk from the Metro. For the first time in almost a year, I walked up the escalator and to the office and didn't get winded. Now that I'm excited about!! THANKS, JJ!

—*Diane W.*

I did great! I lost exactly 15 pounds. My oval face is back, stomach has tightened, skin is clearer and my clothes aren't as tight. Love this cleanse.

—*Michelle D.*

I am down 12 pounds and a uniform size. I have so much energy and less joint pain. This is by far the best cleanse I've ever done. The support from JJ and her team is amazing.

—*Maria D.*

My discipline game has risen to the challenge. I'm so proud of me. I lost 14.3 pounds. I knew results would come if I just committed to do my best and adhere to the guidelines of the cleanse. And it wasn't that hard. My mind was right, the keto smoothies and meals are dee-lish—which makes it very easy to stick with. The Tabata is fun and challenging, and intermittent fasting is going smoothly! I'm so so so proud of me!! I weighed a couple times. I've surpassed my goal for this cleanse, weight wise. But my true goal was to commit, to exercise discipline and show up for myself doing my very best. I DID THAT!!! Yay me!

—*Michelle M.*

I'm feeling good. I lost 13 pounds, stomach flatter, better sleep, and clothes fit better. My well-being is on point. I can feel how the detox and weight loss refreshed my mind, body, and spirit, including the Tabata exercises. I'm grateful for my healthy journey. Thanks, JJ, for all your heart of love.

—*Gwen A.*

I have lost 10.6 pounds and several inches. I love the keto smoothies and meal recipes and will continue for another two weeks. Thanks for the plan, grocery list, and Tabata exercises. I just love it!

—*Shelley A.*

Whoo-hoo! Down almost 10 pounds. My non-scale victories . . . feeling accomplished, much less fatigue, clothes feel roomier. . . . I'm feeling myself a bit.

—*JoAnn W.*

I'm down 12 pounds and lots of inches. I did great. I am going to continue with this plan until I lose all my extra weight.

—*Sandy C.*

I've lost 11 pounds and 3 inches off my waistline but the journey continues for me. . . . I will do the Keto Cleanse until I get to my goal weight! Thanks, JJ Smith.

—*Tasha B.*

I was 290 and am down to 280. I lost 10 pounds in 2 weeks. I thank God for that and I plan to continue until I reach my healthy weight. Thank you, JJ Smith, love you to life.

—*Joyce W.*

I did wonderful. I lost 7 pounds, and my energy is up, my knees feel so much better, inflammation is gone and so are the inches! My clothes let me know that!!! Praise God and thanks to JJ and team!!

—*Linda S.*

I lost 22 pounds so far on the keto cleanse. It feels good to be able to have such high energy. I look down and see my feet instead of belly. This is a good feeling.

—*Robert D.*

I lost 15.5 pounds! I definitely feel less bloated and have more energy. Lost several inches in my waistline. Those Keto Smoothies are on point, finally found some swordfish too! Now I need to do some strength training and toning!

—*Christy L.*

Amazing! I've lost 14 pounds on the New Keto Cleanse. I feel amazing! My clothes fit better and I look better. I completed this New Keto Cleanse with ease. My body needed this after the COVID-19 shutdown. I binged so much junk food during the pandemic. But I'm back on track now!

—*Jessica R.*

Your program is amazing, I got my discipline back, I lost 14 pounds, my energy level is coming along . . . thank you, JJ Smith, for this new lifestyle. It is a winner! I'm looking forward to continuing those meals. My family loved them!

—*Tammi A.*

I am down 17 pounds. I was really strict on this cleanse. I measured every meal because of my busy life. I didn't work out every day, but I am happy with the results and hoping to do it again soon. Thank you, JJ Smith. You really outdid yourself with this one. This keto cleanse is my new favorite!

—*Lisa A.*

Thirteen pounds on day 14!! Unfortunately, I did not measure myself before but my clothes are definitely looser. My energy and discipline have been so good! I plan to keep following intermittent fasting and low carb/low sugar! I have more energy with it!

—*Shelly C.*

I've learned so much discipline during this cleanse and intermittent fasting has been a game changer for me. I don't have any more cravings for sweets thanks either. I still have some work to do but the progress so far is worth it. I'm not huffing and puffing with my daughter asking, "Why you breathing so hard?" That's progress!!

—*Mary T.*

I said my scale is broken! LOL. But really, I've lost so much weight and mostly inches. I've been able to get in some jeans that I refuse to get rid of because they are so nice. I got in them with room to spare. Thank you for giving both me and my husband another way to live this beautiful life.

—*Pam M.*

Good morning! I lost 9 pounds and OMG tons of inches. I don't feel sluggish in the morning. I feel so good right now!

—*Denise E.*

My energy is so much better. I feel alert. I lost 11 pounds but more inches than pounds. I've lost 2.5 inches from my stomach, 2 inches from my hips. I forgot to measure my arms but my shirts are a lot looser!! I'm definitely feeling more determined to continue with this keto/low carb transition. I'm over 50 and processed carbs are not my friend. LOL.

—*Arlene B.*

Down 10.7 pounds! I am so happy with my progress. I could've done better with Tabata and drinking more water so I will work on that. I'm getting married so this Cleanse was right on time. I surprised myself and did better with intermittent fasting than I thought I would. I used to love big breakfasts so that was a big adjustment but I did it!

—*Randy D.*

I am down 9.2 pounds. I wish I took my measurements because I know I lost a lot of inches too. Before COVID, I recently bought a new waist trainer because the one I had was too big. I tried it on the day of the cleanse and it could not fit. In two weeks, I now can get into the third hook. I lost that many inches. How great is that. I will continue this keto cleanse for sure. I just need to up my water intake. The water was making me a bit bloated but it's getting better. I did Tabata every day but one. I'm glad my body is finally detoxing.

—*Tracie C.*

My brother and I both lost 10 pounds. I noticed that I have wayyy more energy, my clothes feel looser, and my skin is glowing. Literally glowing, I just feel better in general. I stuck to the meal plan and really enjoyed the meals and keto smoothies.

—*Tia R.*

Lost 10 pounds. Energy level is great! Worked out every day and averaged over 10K steps a day. My waist is trimming down. My clothes fit better and the food has been delicious! Will need to drink more water this week!

—*Lisa J.*

So far I'm 12 pounds down and my husband is 11 pounds down! It's just the beginning for both of us! I know I've lost inches too because my clothes are fitting loose. My energy is way up!

—Debbie S.

Released 8.2 pounds and feeling motivated to keep pushing forward! I'm feeling amazing and lost 4 inches off my thighs. So proud of myself. My energy is off the charts and I feel great!

—Capri T.

I lost 8 pounds on the Cleanse, and my waist beads are falling. I'm proud of this and I will continue this program daily. I would have done better but one too many cheat meals. But I'll do better next time.

—Sherrie B.

I'm fitting in jeans that I couldn't before the Cleanse. I'm so much lighter. I feel the lightness and see it. I mostly like how being on this Keto Cleanse put me back in the mindset of preparing my meals, and I loved the variety of food choices.

—Nina D.

Down 8 pounds . . . starting round two tomorrow . . . adjusted to intermittent fasting . . . best plan I've ever tried and will continue with the recipes. I loved them. Thank you, JJ.

—Allison C.

Down 9 pounds. The food was delicious!! I could have done better on my water intake and Tabata, but I will do better the next time. I'm feeling amazing. This has been the most fun and most delicious food eating cleanse I've ever tried.

—*Carolyn E.*

I lost 12 pounds and I feel fabulous. This was such an awesome journey. I drank my water and ate the delicious meals. I was not hungry at all on this journey. Even my family enjoyed the meals and asked me to make their favorites again. This Keto Cleanse is something I can stick with. I will continue to follow this program. Thank you so much, JJ.

—*Kim S.*

After two weeks, I lost 15 pounds. My starting weight was 173 and after gaining a few pounds back, I am still down to 158 pounds. I have more energy and look and feel great! I'm surprised how much I enjoyed this.

—*Dana S.*

Feeling great, no achy joints, smooth skin, full of energy, broke my 10-pound plateau, and lost a lot of inches. I will continue this low-carb/low-sugar lifestyle and continue on with the keto cleanse. I feel so great. This will definitely be my everyday life.

—*Stephanie C.*

I lost 11 pounds in the first 10 days and many inches off my waist. I haven't done my final 14 day weigh-in yet. I know this Cleanse works if you stick with it. My family told me I look so much younger and prettier!

—*Janelle T.*

I did not get a chance to weigh or do my measurements but my energy is better than it's been in awhile. I don't feel sluggish. I've stayed the course and I'm proud of myself. I feel too good to not continue this Cleanse. Plus the jeans I jumped five times to put on a couple weeks ago, I only jumped once to get in this week. I am winning!

—*Rhonda W.*

I've lost 14.7 pounds and my discipline was on point! It was easy to stick with this keto cleanse. This is by far my most favorite one and I've done all of them. I'm actually going to continue beyond day 14 and do this plan every single day. Thank you, JJ!!! This has been AMAZING!

—*Janice R.*

As James Brown says: I feel good! I finished and I am so proud of myself, I lost 10 pounds and I do have more energy. I will be continuing for another 14 days, this is now my new lifestyle. I finally found something I can do for life, thank you, JJ.

—*Shanae J.*

Well it's official, I'm a size 12 again! My husband said I was thicker than a Snickers. So, it's safe to say I lost two dress sizes! I feel so much better in my clothes now!

—*Elena E.*

I've lost 12 pounds and not sure how many inches (wish I had measured myself) but my pants are falling off. A family member that hasn't seen me since I started the cleanse noticed a big difference too. Here's to a lifetime of eating healthier! I love this keto cleanse!

—*Roberta D.*

I'm 73 years old so any seniors wondering if you can, yes you can and yes you should! The keto cleanse transformed my life. I am down 13 pounds and several inches. I have eaten foods I never had before and fixed them in ways I never would have thought of. This 73-year-old grandma is full of energy and rocking it!

—*Janet C.*

This keto cleanse completely gave me life! The only weight-loss regimen that has ever worked for me has been the 10-Day Green Smoothie Cleanse, but I must admit I started to get bored with it and I couldn't stay focused. This keto cleanse restored my faith, and I've been so excited to try the new recipes each day and I completely love it! Down 12 pounds, more energy, motivation, and focus! I will not stop and will keep going!

—*Missy L.*

The meals are amazing but my appetite has gone downhill, I'm not even hungry. My energy level is off the hook and most of all I'm sleeping so much better. My joint pain is much more manageable. And I'm down 8 pounds and 2 inches off my waist.

—*Eva J.*

I am down 14 pounds and many inches. My back fat is vanishing, and so far I am able to stick to the plan without any cheating. I didn't do the Tabata exercises but I walked from time to time. I really loved my results!

—*Carrie D.*

I'm down 10 pounds and feeling great! My pants are not as tight as they were before the cleanse. My sleep has improved and I have less knee pain. I was so inspired by this group and all the support that has been shown to keep me motivated not to quit. My birthday is next month, and my plan is to continue with the keto cleanse as a lifestyle. I will allow myself the grace not to be perfect as I continue my journey. Thank You, JJ and the Green Smoothie Family!

—*Catherine G.*

After the first week, I was down nearly 8 pounds. By the end of the second week, I was down 14 pounds. I am loving the low-carb keto recipes and the keto smoothies make it even better. I AM ADDICTED TO TABATA WORKOUTS!!!! Thank you, JJ!

—*Tosha M.*

I haven't weighed myself yet, but the proof is in my clothes. My neck, shoulders, arms, and thighs are all thinner. I'm sleeping better and not unconsciously eating. I feel in control of my eating habits. I will continue the keto cleanse forever.

—*Brenda J.*

I am down 11 pounds, and I feel the inches lost in my clothes. I have mega energy and my skin is smooth and glowing. This was by far my favorite cleanse, and so I am continuing this as my new lifestyle. Next goal is to get more water and exercise in on a consistent basis.

—Denise L.

I lost 9 pounds and I really love this keto challenge because I'm not sitting here counting the days for it to be over. In my opinion, it was much easier than the 10-Day Green Smoothie Cleanse. I enjoyed the meals and the keto smoothies. It didn't feel like a diet. I did not feel deprived at all. This is something I really enjoyed!

—Veronica R.

I was not consistent with my eating, but I still lost 6 pounds and 1 inch off my waist. My energy has improved. It was easy because I cheated a lot and still got great results for two weeks' time.

—Carrie M.

I survived it (my number one goal) and 12 pounds down—my liver is refreshed, I'm hydrated and sugar levels getting back to normal. My NSV—no alcohol consumption (it was a daily thing), no eating junk food, regained so much self-control. I did some movement and was fairly consistent with meal planning and prep. I'm proud of myself.

—Doris P.

I feel good, amazing, and alive. I got on the scale this morning and I was down 11.4 pounds. I am pleased and feeling myself. I can finally see my ankles and kneecaps!!

—Irene F.

I've lost 12 pounds and my blood pressure is amazing. A couple nights I slipped a little and ate a small amount of carbs. I've lost quite a few inches in the waist, stomach, and upper back. I can't go without a belt, which was on the last hole, but three holes are back now. I'm going shopping for bras soon; they're now too loose. I feel great. I'm in to win this time. Thanks for everything you do for this group and all the support, JJ.

—Yolanda S.

My discipline has been great. Energy is decent. I have been battling thyroid problems for 20 years! But I was still able to lose 8 pounds, 1.5 inches in my bust, 1.5 inches in my waist, and 2.5 inches in my hips! My husband lost 14 pounds! We loved this keto cleanse.

—Michelle M.

I have a slimmer waistline. I am proud of myself. I will continue this journey because I love me and am thankful for the new way of keto eating. I have 6 pounds to my goal weight, and I will achieve it within the next two weeks on this keto cleanse. Thanks to all the ladies and big thank you to JJ Smith for an awesome program.

—Esther L.

I'm so excited. I'm down 15.8 pounds after the 14 days and feel great!

—*Kimberley H.*

I'm feeling awesome! Lost 11 pounds—as well as many inches. Love the new habits and discipline! Intermittent fasting is really nice! I'm so happy I dramatically cut down on my sugar intake. I am so surprised I made it through without a struggle, and my stomach has gotten so much smaller.

—*Candy E.*

CHAPTER 11

Conclusion

Congrats! You're ready to take back control of your health and weight. You are now fully equipped with the knowledge to lose weight more effortlessly and keep it off long-term. It's only two weeks, but you have the ability to change your habits, body, and life by committing to being consistent for that time.

Be sure to journal and take pictures. You need to take pictures so you can observe your progress from week to week. Journaling will help you write down how you're feeling and how the supplements are affecting your health and moods. You need to be aware of exactly what is working well for you and what is not.

The body is fully capable of healing, rejuvenating, and restoring itself to optimum health, and the 14-Day New Keto Cleanse allows you to do just that. After the fourteen days, you will experience great health benefits. You will naturally slim down. You will begin to think more clearly. You will feel energized and more alive. You will notice a clearer complexion. You will feel happier and more balanced. You will have the motivation to continue on your health and weight-loss journey.

If you prepare your mind and absorb the knowledge offered to you in this book, you will have all the power you need to become your best self and transform your life in every way. Embrace the journey! Stay focused until the end of the two weeks. Follow the program day in and day out and be consistent. I wish you much success and happiness on your journey!

In closing, I want to leave you with my *Ten Commandments for Looking Young and Feeling Great*, which I always share at the end of my books.

Thou shalt love thyself. Self-love is essential to survival. There is no successful, authentic relationship with others without self-love. We cannot water the land from a dry well. Self-love is not selfish or self-indulgent. We have to take care of our needs first so we can give to others from abundance.

Thou shalt take responsibility for thine own health and well-being. If you want to be healthy, have more energy, and feel great, you must take the time to learn what is involved and apply it to your own life. You have to watch what goes into your mouth, how much exercise and physical activity you get, and what thoughts you're thinking throughout the day.

Thou shalt sleep. Sleep is the body's way of recharging the system. Sleep is the easiest yet most underrated activity for healing the body. Lack of sleep definitely saps your glow and instantly ages you, giving you puffy red eyes with dark circles under them.

Thou shalt detoxify and cleanse the body. Detoxifying the body means ridding the body of poisons and toxins so that you can speed up weight loss and restore great health. A clean body is a beautiful body!

Thou shalt remember that a healthy body is a sexy body. Real women's bodies look beautiful! It's about getting healthy and having style and confidence and wearing clothes that match your body type.

Thou shalt eat healthy, natural, whole foods. Healthy eating can turn back the hands of time and return the body to a more youthful state. When you eat natural foods, you simply look and feel better. You keep the body clean at the cellular level and look radiant despite your age. Eating healthy should be part of your "beauty regimen."

Thou shalt embrace healthy aging. The goal is not to stop the aging process but to embrace it. Healthy aging is staying healthy as you age, looking and feeling great despite your age.

Thou shalt commit to a lifestyle change. Losing weight permanently requires a commitment to changes . . . in your thinking, your lifestyle, your mindset. It requires gaining knowledge and making permanent changes in your life for the better!

Thou shalt embrace the journey. This is a journey that will change your life. It's not a diet but rather a lifestyle! Be kind and supportive to yourself. Learn to applaud yourself for the smallest accomplishment. And when you slip up sometimes, know that it is okay. It is called being human.

Thou shalt live, love, and laugh. Laughter is still good for the soul. Live your life with passion! Never give up on your dreams! And most important . . . love! Remember that love never fails!

Now that you have experienced the power of the 14-Day New Keto Cleanse, be sure to share your success story with others and help them to reclaim their health and life.

Appendix: JJ's Top Ten Favorite Detox Methods

Detoxifying the body and eliminating toxins can be accomplished through various detoxification methods. (I describe twenty-one ways to detox the body for weight loss and overall health in my book *Green Smoothies for Life*.) However, I want to highlight my top ten favorite detox methods that I do quite often.

Everyone's toxic overload is different, and many factors come into play, such as your health status, weight, metabolism, age, and genetics. If you want to enhance your detoxification and cleansing, here are my top ten favorite ways to detox the body to support the cleansing process during or after the 14-Day New Keto Cleanse:

Alkaline water

Body brushing

Castor oil packs

Colon cleansing

Detox foot bath/foot pads

Detox water (ACV
 detox water)

Epsom salt baths

Green smoothies

Liver cleansing

Saunas

Bonus: Whole body
vibration

Alkaline Water

It is important to stay hydrated, especially when fasting and dieting. Dehydration can lead to unclear thinking, mood changes, bloating, and constipation. Water is involved in every type of cellular process in the body. So, if you're dehydrated, all of these processes run less efficiently, including your metabolism. By getting enough water, you regulate how much you eat as well as help the body digest food properly. A study published in *Obesity* found that overweight adults who drank sixteen ounces of water thirty minutes before their meals lost nine more pounds at the end of a twelve-week period than those who didn't drink any water before meals. Ideally, you should drink half your body weight in ounces. For example, if you weigh two hundred pounds, you should be drinking one hundred ounces of water daily.

My favorite type of water that enhances hydration is alkaline water. Alkaline water has a higher pH level (8 or 9) than regular drinking water (6 or 7). The pH level measures how acidic or alkaline a substance is on a scale of 0 to 14. For example, something with a pH of 1 would be very acidic, and something with a pH of 13 or 14 would be very alkaline. Your overall pH balance is extremely important to determining good health. The goal is a healthy state of alkalinity. Many experts say that disease cannot exist when the body is in an alkaline state. When the body is in an acidic state, the body is not healthy. An acidic body puts you at a greater risk for all kinds of disease, chronic illness, and weight gain. Drinking alkaline water (ion water or hydrogen-rich water) can help to keep the body in an alkaline state, detoxify the body, increase energy levels, and leave the skin looking smoother, more elastic, and more youthful.

A simple way to make your water more alkaline is to add a squeeze of lemon or lime (which, after going through the digestive process, creates alkaline by-products) to a glass of distilled water. It's important to use distilled water because tap water may have additives or artificial ingredients. You can also purchase pH drops and add them to your water as another way to make it more alkaline.

You can also buy alkaline water in health food stores or get a portable alkaline water bottle that converts regular water to alkaline water. A more expensive option is to buy a machine that converts the water from your faucet to alkaline water—for example, a Kangen machine.

It is recommended that you not drink alkaline water with meals, but any other times throughout the day are fine. You need to build up how much alkaline water your body can handle, beginning with about eight ounces a day. If you drink too much alkaline water too quickly, you will get strong detox symptoms, such as headaches or rashes. Work your way up slowly until you use alkaline water as your primary water to meet your daily water-intake goals.

Body Brushing

Body brushing (also known as dry brushing) is done with a natural boar-bristle or Tampico brush, which can be found in health food stores, Whole Foods, or Trader Joe's, or on Amazon. Dry brushing on a regular basis lightens the burden on the liver by helping to remove excess waste in the body. Dry brushing stimulates the lymphatic system, which is a secondary circulatory system underneath the skin that rids the body of toxic wastes, bacteria, and dead cells. By body brushing, you move the toxins along and out of the body for elimination. By brushing the body from head to toe with the dry brush—focusing on the lymphatic drainage regions, like behind the knee—you'll improve the efficiency of the whole lymphatic system.

Firm, gentle brushstrokes across the skin will improve your blood circulation, clean out clogged pores, and enable your body to remove toxins faster. Body brushing removes dead skin layers and encourages cell renewal for smoother skin. If the liver is a fat-burning organ, then the lymph system can be called a fat-processing system. Cleansing the liver and lymphatic system are key to weight loss.

Further, increasing circulation to the skin could reduce the appearance of cellulite, which is just toxic material accumulated in your body's fat cells.

Directions for Body Brushing

First remove your clothes and start on dry skin before bathing.
Begin brushing the soles of the feet.
Next, brush from the ankles to the calves, concentrating on
     the area behind the knees, using long, firm, upward strokes

toward the heart. The lymphatic fluid flows through the body toward the heart, so it's important that you brush in the same direction.

Your back is the only exception to the rule above; brush from the neck down to the lower back.

Then brush from the knees to the groin, the thighs, and the buttocks.

If you're a woman, make circular strokes around your thighs and buttocks to help mobilize fat stores, such as cellulite.

Then brush the torso, avoiding the breasts.

Finally, make long strokes from the wrists to the shoulders and underarms.

Never brush over inflamed skin, open sores, sunburned skin, or skin tumors.

The entire process should take no more than three to five minutes and will leave your skin feeling totally invigorated.

Make sure to shower to wash away the dead skin cells and impurities. Then follow with a natural moisturizer of your choice, such as coconut oil.

The best times to brush are in the morning before showering or at night before you go to bed.

Castor Oil Packs

Castor oil packs are typically used by naturopaths to help stimulate and detoxify the liver. Some find they really help decongest the liver and minimize bloating and fluid retention. A castor oil pack is placed directly on the skin to increase circulation and promote elimination and healing of the tissues and organs underneath the skin. It is used to stimulate the liver, relieve pain, increase lymphatic circulation, reduce inflammation, and improve digestion. Castor oil appears to work by drawing blood circulation and biological energy to the area where it is applied and then drawing toxins out of the body.

Castor oil packs are made by soaking pieces of cotton or wool flannel in castor oil and placing them on the abdomen, especially over the liver. The flannel is covered with a sheet of plastic wrap, and a hot water bottle or heating pad is placed over the plastic to heat the pack. You keep the pack on for thirty to forty-five minutes while in a relaxed position and rest. After removing the pack, cleanse the area with a solution of water and baking soda. Store the pack in a covered container in the refrigerator. Each pack may be reused up to thirty times. It's generally recommended that a castor oil pack be used for three to seven days in one week as a detoxification treatment. You can also try sleeping with the castor oil pack overnight as well for increased benefit.

You can place the cloth on the right side of the abdomen to stimulate the liver or directly on inflamed and swollen joints and muscle strains. It can be used on the abdomen to relieve constipation and other digestive disorders and on the lower abdomen in cases of menstrual irregularities and uterine and ovarian cysts.

Castor oil should not be taken internally. It should not be applied to broken skin or used during pregnancy, breastfeeding, or menstrual flow.

Colon Cleansing

Periodic colon cleansing cleans the colon by removing waste that may be stuck along the colon walls. This excess waste can produce toxins that enter the bloodstream and cause various symptoms, including bloating, gas, fatigue, acne, and belly fat.

One way to cleanse the colon is with herbs and supplements taken in the form of powders or capsules. Cleansing the colon with herbs or supplements can help expel its contents and draw out old fecal matter. You can find colon-cleansing supplements online or in health food stores, supermarkets, or drugstores.

One of the main theories behind colon cleansing is the belief that undigested foods can cause mucus buildup in the colon. This buildup produces toxins, which enter the blood's circulation, poisoning the body. Thus, colon cleansing will clear toxins from the body or neutralize them and clear out excess mucus and congestion.

A nice benefit of colon cleansing is the reduction of constipation. A poor diet that deprives someone of essential nutrients can cause the intestinal walls to become lined with a plaque-like substance that is not healthy. Colon cleansing not only helps remove the junk from intestinal walls, it also allows waste to pass more freely. The other noticeable benefit is the elimination of diarrhea, which is normally caused by toxins and can cause problems for the whole process of solidifying the waste.

Look at Your Poop

A good way to evaluate your health is to check your poop. As an example, bowel movements (BMs) that are black or reddish indicate potential health problems. Thin BMs suggest that more fiber is needed in the diet or that there is some type of imbalance in the digestive tract. If you have chronic constipation and your BMs are rock solid, this may be an indication that your liver is overworked.

If you experience chronic constipation or difficult bowel movements for an extended period of time, you should seek medical advice.

Your bowel movements will help you understand what's going on with your body. Healthy bowel movements have the following characteristics:

- Occur one to three times a day, definitely no less than once per day.
- Should not have a strong, foul odor.
- Should be medium brown in color, shaped like a banana, about the width of a sausage.
- Should float, not sink right to the bottom of the toilet.

A very powerful and effective colon cleanser that I've used for overnight results is a magnesium-oxygen supplement. It combines magnesium oxide compounds that have been ozonated and stabilized to release oxygen throughout the entire digestive system over twelve hours or more. The magnesium acts as a vehicle to transport oxygen throughout the body and has the gentle effect of loosening toxins and acidic waste and transporting them out of the body. Oxygen also supports the growth of friendly bacteria, which is essential for proper digestive and intestinal health.

Magnesium-oxygen supplements are safe for regular use, but I would recommend they always be used during heavy detoxification and fasting periods to help keep the colon clean and increase bowel activity. I offer my favorite brand on my website at www.JJSmithOnline.com. Folks have experienced decreased bloating, gas, and constipation with the product. However, for me, it's knowing that I'm eliminating toxins and waste from my entire digestive tract that provides the biggest benefit.

For intensive colon cleansing, magnesium-oxygen supplements taken for seven to ten days are an effective way to jumpstart any weight-loss program. They are safe for regular use and can also be used on a longer-term basis for daily, ongoing detoxification. In contrast to synthetic laxatives like senna, a quality magnesium-oxygen supplement is non-habit-forming and actually strengthens all organ functions, making it a safe long-term option.

As always, check with your doctor and be sure to follow the directions on the label. For most people, anywhere from three to five supplements taken at bedtime for seven to ten days will provide an effective digestive cleansing. If you experience loose stools or other side effects, simply reduce the dosage and be sure to take the supplement just once a day, at bedtime. And please watch the stool to see what comes out. You will be amazed and possibly disgusted.

Detox Foot Pads/Foot Baths
Detox foot pads
This just might be the easiest detox method of them all. Detox foot pads are a quick and easy way to rid the body of toxins.

They are like large white bandages that have a variety of ingredients and herbs that help the body draw out toxins, even heavy metals and poisons. You put them on the bottoms of your feet overnight, held on by adhesive strips. In the morning, you discard them. They are helpful with aches, pains, sore muscles, joint pains, swelling, and bloating.

Detox foot pads use the same philosophy as acupuncture, as the foot contains more than sixty acupuncture points. When blood circulates through the foot, the detox foot pad utilizes these acupuncture points to draw out toxins. As toxins are pulled from the tissues and cells in the body, they end up in the feet, where they can be eliminated with the detox foot pad.

My favorite brands are BodyRelief Foot Pads and Asako Detox Foot Pads, which really help me with joint aches and pains.

Detox foot baths

The detox foot bath (ionic foot bath), found in many salons and spas, works by soaking your feet in a warm saltwater solution made up of many different toxin-drawing ingredients. An ionic detox foot bath is a natural method of assisting the body in eliminating harmful toxins and heavy metals. The ionic activity in the water shoots through your body fat and draws the toxins out through the hundreds of pores in your feet. Thirty minutes is the average time for a detox foot bath, which costs a little more than the foot pads ($60 versus $15). A detox foot bath is said to make joint movement easier in the knees and elbows. It's an alternative medicine option for people who suffer from headaches and chronic joint and bone pain.

A detox foot bath is very simple and extremely relaxing. It is typically offered as a spa service under the name of Aqua Chi Foot Bath.

Detox Water (ACV Detox Water)

Drinking apple cider vinegar (ACV) diluted with water one to three times a day is an easy and effective way to detoxify and improve digestion. ACV has great cleansing properties due to its rich content of minerals, vitamins, and enzymes. It helps the body remove toxins and waste more efficiently before they have time to accumulate and damage the body. ACV is known to aid digestion and improve bowel movements. It also helps to detoxify the liver, purify the blood, and improve circulation due to its powerful enzymes that break down bad cholesterol and prevent it from clogging your arteries.

ACV stimulates your metabolism and makes you burn fat faster. Because ACV stimulates digestion, it also reduces the amount of time fats remain in the digestive tract. If fats are present longer than necessary during digestion, more fat will be absorbed by the body.

If you are going to use ACV for weight loss, you need to drink it first thing every morning. You can drink it up to three times per day—before each meal—to accelerate results.

The recipe I like consists of the following:

2 tablespoons raw unfiltered apple cider vinegar
6 to 8 ounces water
Squeeze of lemon
Dash cayenne pepper

(You can add stevia to taste but it's not necessary.)

My favorite brands of ACV are Bragg and WhiteHouse.

Epsom Salt Baths

Epsom salt is rich in both magnesium and sulfate. Magnesium and sulfate can be easily absorbed through the skin. In an Epsom salt detox bath, the magnesium sulfate is absorbed through the skin, which helps to draw out toxins, extra fluid, and cellular waste from the body. By drawing out the excess fluid in your body, Epsom salt baths help to eliminate bloating and excess water weight. In fact, celebrities often use Epsom salt baths two to three days before a big event so that they look their absolute best.

To make an Epsom salt bath: Start slowly by adding one tablespoon of Epsom salt to your bath water. Gradually, over time and several baths, increase the amount of salt to two cups. If you start with big quantities without a gentle introduction first, you might suffer some adverse symptoms, like extreme fatigue. Soak in the bath for fifteen to twenty minutes and unwind. Don't stay in the bath for longer than twenty-five minutes or you might end up exhausting yourself. Be sure to rehydrate well during and after your hot bath. Epsom salt baths can be done once or twice per week.

To provide even more benefit, you can add ten drops of the following essential oils, which will help with various conditions:

Lavender: calming and relaxation
Cedarwood: depression and mood swings
Peppermint: fatigue
Chamomile and rosemary: headaches

Green Smoothies

Green smoothies have such a powerful ability to detox the body, they deserve a category all by themselves. Green smoothies give your body the quality nutrition it needs while cleansing your cells and insides. Vitamins, minerals, and other nutrients will be absorbed by your body more efficiently, allowing your cells to become like new as you begin to look and feel younger.

Green smoothies are filled with chlorophyll, which is similar in structure to the hemoglobin in human blood. So every time you drink a green smoothie, it's like receiving a blood transfusion. They are a powerful cleansing method for the body.

As I referenced at the beginning of this section, once your body has utilized nutrients from the food you consume, it disposes of the unused food particles and waste produced by the digestive process. If you don't properly and completely eliminate undigested food, whatever remains backs up and leaves toxins and waste in your body. But thanks to green smoothies, you can get the fiber you need to cleanse your body, tone your digestive system, and eliminate toxins.

My favorite types of green smoothies are keto smoothies, which are keto-friendly green smoothies that are lower in sugar and carbs than traditional green smoothies. In this book, I've provided my favorite keto smoothie recipes that are delicious and creamy with all the nutritional benefits of green smoothies to help you detox, reduce cravings, and lose weight in just fourteen days.

Liver Cleansing

The secret to losing weight and keeping it off is to keep the liver healthy and operating at peak performance. The liver is the number-one secret weapon to weight loss. The liver is responsible for breaking down, eliminating, and neutralizing toxins in the body and breaking down fats in the body. Therefore, it is essential that we cleanse the liver to improve the body's detoxification capabilities and to help the body metabolize and burn fats.

Although there are several organs of elimination in the body, most health practitioners agree that the liver is the primary one. It has been said that the length and quality of life depends on proper liver function. The liver works day and night to cleanse the blood of toxins such as unhealthy chemicals, bad bacteria, and other foreign substances. The liver is also responsible for breaking down fats in the body. It is critical to keep the liver clean and healthy and working at peak performance.

When your liver functions efficiently, it is much easier for you to lose weight. The liver has to perform well enough to eliminate the toxins that are causing fat cells in the body. If you have body-fat accumulation, especially around the waist and midsection (i.e., belly fat), it suggests that your liver may not be functioning properly or as efficiently as it could. To lose this excess weight, you have to detoxify and cleanse the liver, which leads to not only a slimmer waistline but also a thinner body.

The most common liver disease in America is a condition known as fatty liver disease, in which the liver stops processing fat and begins storing it right around the waistline. The main characteristic of fatty liver disease is too much fat stored in liver cells. In the United States, fatty liver disease affects eighty to one hundred million adults. The major cause of fatty liver disease is overconsumption of sugar, high-fructose corn syrup, and refined carbohydrates (like white flour, white rice, and white sugar).

Our skin, sleep, moods, energy, and longevity all depend on the liver's ability to function optimally. The great news is that the liver is resilient and can easily regenerate itself. Even if you cut off a piece of the liver, the organ will regrow and continue to function.

One easy way to cleanse the liver is to take herbs or supplements, such as milk thistle, dandelion root, and burdock. These herbs are all-natural and very effective at liver detoxification. My favorite liver detox supplement is one I created called Liver Focus, which can be found on www.JJSmithOnline.com. There are other products that may use only one herb, like milk thistle, but Liver Focus is so much more powerful because it is a combination of seven herbs. Liver Focus also has additional ingredients for weight loss. Other brands focus on removing toxins for liver health, but Liver Focus focuses on removing toxins and accelerating fat burning in the body.

Follow a liver-cleansing routine for several months until fat burning increases in the body. Additionally, you may notice that the symptoms of a sluggish liver improve.

Symptoms of a sluggish liver include the following:

Belly fat or fat around the abdomen
Sclera (white part of the eye) no longer white
Poor skin tone, including acne or breakouts around the nose, cheeks, and chin
Dark circles under the eyes
Yellow-coated tongue

Bitter taste in the mouth
Headaches
Moodiness and irritability

Completing a liver cleanse can be a positive and rejuvenating experience that yields numerous health benefits. As you improve liver health, you increase your body's ability to detoxify itself, improve its fat-burning capabilities, and achieve optimum health.

Saunas

A sauna session helps you sweat out toxins, burn calories, and come out with glowing skin. It also boosts the immune system and relaxes the muscles. So many benefits!

The skin is the largest organ of elimination for the body. Perspiring through the skin flushes out toxins and impurities. Additionally, the heat of the sauna causes the body's temperature to rise, which can help kill any virus, bacteria, fungus, or parasite in the body.

A sauna session can do more to clean, detoxify, and simply freshen your skin than anything else. The heat from the sauna opens up the pores of the skin, allowing impurities and toxins to flush themselves out of the body. It hydrates and moisturizes the skin and is particularly beneficial to people with dry skin. One of my clients found that by sweating out her toxins in the sauna, her acne cleared up; this was due to her sweating out the toxins as opposed to them being released through the skin, causing acne and other rashes.

A sauna session will speed up metabolism, which in turn results in weight loss. You can burn three hundred to five hundred calories in fifteen to twenty minutes in a sauna, equivalent to one to two hours of brisk walking or one hour of aerobic exercise. Most people sit in a sauna for fifteen to thirty minutes, and rarely longer than forty-five minutes.

The high temperature of the sauna causes an artificial fever, which sends a "wake-up call" to the immune system and increases the white blood cell count.

The heat also warms and relaxes tense muscles. This relaxation helps to reduce stress levels, revive mental clarity, and improve overall physical and emotional health.

The best type of sauna is an infrared sauna, which produces what is known as radiant heat. The heat of an infrared sauna also penetrates more deeply without the discomfort and draining effect often experienced in a conventional steam sauna. An infrared sauna produces two to three times more sweat volume, and due to the lower temperatures used (110°F to 130°F), it is considered a safer alternative for those at cardiovascular risk. It accelerates the removal of toxic wastes lodged in the fatty tissues. The sweating caused by deep heat helps eliminate dead skin cells and improve skin tone and elasticity. The heat produced in infrared saunas is extremely helpful for various skin conditions, including acne, eczema, and cellulite. Plus, studies have shown that you can burn six hundred calories in thirty minutes in an infrared sauna.

I enjoy sitting in the sauna several times a week because it has both health benefits and beauty benefits.

Cautions:

The sauna can be dehydrating, so it is important to drink lots of water before and after your session.

If you have heart issues, particularly sensitive skin or asthma, or if you are pregnant, you should not sit in a sauna until you have checked with your doctor.

BONUS: Whole Body Vibration

You may not have even heard of it yet, but whole-body vibration (WBV) is the exercise of the future. The WBV machine uses a vibrating plate that you stand on for ten to fifteen minutes, causing rapid muscle contractions that burn calories and provide you with muscle strength that you could otherwise get by working out for an hour in the gym. However, WBV involves no sweating or discomfort and leaves you feeling rejuvenated, calmer, and slimmer.

Many of the world's best athletes in the NFL, NHL, NBA, and Olympic sports, as well as Hollywood celebrities, are using WBV to lose weight, build muscle tone and bone density, relieve back pain and arthritis, improve circulation, and speed up metabolism. As a woman, I've found it to be especially beneficial for burning fat and cellulite around the thighs, hips, and buttocks.

The stimulation of whole-body vibration exercise delivers quick results that are simple yet phenomenal. WBV puts the muscles in a situation where they must expand and contract continually at a rapid rate, about twenty-five to fifty times per second, which helps to strengthen them. These contractions pump extra oxygen into the cells, which allows them to repair and regenerate quickly, resulting in amazing body transformations. Keep in mind, though, that maximum fat burning and weight loss is accomplished through WBV only when combined with proper nutrition.

The muscle contractions caused by a vibration plate will probably not build as much muscle mass as lifting weights, but unless you're a body builder, it is still very effective for maintaining muscle tone and strength.

There are two main types of WBV machines, those that vibrate up and down using a piston-like motion (lineal) and others that vibrate from side to side like an oscillating teeter-totter (pivotal). I have used both, and my personal preference is the pivotal machines. Both machines are effective, but you should research both types if you're interested in starting a WBV routine.

You can also target muscle groups by moving to different positions on the vibration machine to get even faster muscle-building results. Vibration machines are all the rage among celebrities and top athletes whose livelihood depends on their bodies being in top condition, yet they are too busy to spend hours sweating in a gym.

JJ Smith's Bio

www.**JJSmithOnline**.com

JJ Smith is a number-one *New York Times* bestselling author, nutritionist, and certified weight-loss expert, passionate relationship/life coach, and inspirational speaker. She has been featured on *Steve Harvey*, *The Dr. Oz Show*, *The View*, *Rachael Ray*, *The Jamie Foxx Radio Show*, and *The Michael Baisden Show*. JJ has made appearances on NBC, FOX, CBS, and the CW Network, as well as in the pages of *Glamour*, *Essence*, *Heart & Soul*, and *Ladies' Home Journal*. Since reclaiming her health, losing weight, and discovering a "second youth" in her forties, JJ has become a voice of inspiration to those who want to lose weight, be healthy, and get their sexy back. She provides lifestyle solutions for losing weight, getting healthy, looking younger, and improving your love life!

JJ has dedicated her life to the field of healthy eating and living. Her passion is to educate others and share with them the natural remedies to stay slim, restore health, and look and feel younger. JJ has studied many philosophies of natural healing and learned from some of the great teachers of our time. After studying and applying knowledge about how to heal the body and lose weight, JJ went on to receive several certifications—one as a certified nutritionist and another as a certified weight-management expert. She received her certification as nutritionist from the International Institute of Holistic Healing, and her certification as a weight-management specialist from the National Exercise and Sports Trainers Association (NESTA). She is also a member of the American Nutrition Association (ANA).

JJ is the author of the number-one *New York Times* bestseller *The 10-Day Green Smoothie Cleanse*, which is a proven plan to safely and quickly detoxify the body and jump-start weight loss. Most people who follow the plan experience weight loss of up to fifteen pounds in only ten days. JJ is also the author of the *New York Times* bestsellers *Green Smoothies for Life* and *7-Day Apple Cider Vinegar Cleanse*. JJ is also the author of the number-one bestseller *Lose Weight Without Dieting or Working Out!*, a revolutionary system that teaches proven methods for permanent weight loss that anyone can follow, no matter their size, income level, or educational level. And the end result is a healthy, sexy, slim body.

JJ holds a BA in mathematics from Hampton University in Virginia. She continued her education by completing the Wharton Business School Executive Management Certificate program. She also served as vice president and partner in an IT consulting firm, Intact Technology, Inc., in Greenbelt, Maryland. JJ was also the youngest African American to attain a vice president position at a Fortune 500 company. Her hobbies include reading, writing, and deejaying.